THE CLINICAL PSYCHIATRY OF LATE LIFE

BY

FELIX POST

M.D., F.R.C.P., D.P.M.
Physician, The Bethlem Royal Hospital and the
Maudsley Hospital, London

PERGAMON PRESS
OXFORD · LONDON · EDINBURGH · NEW YORK
PARIS · FRANKFURT

Pergamon Press Ltd., Headington Hill Hall, Oxford
4 & 5 Fitzroy Square, London W.1

Pergamon Press (Scotland) Ltd., 2 & 3 Teviot Place, Edinburgh 1

Pergamon Press Inc., 122 East 55th Street, New York 22, N.Y.

Pergamon Press GmbH, Kaiserstrasse 75, Frankfurt-am-Main

Federal Publications Ltd., Times House, River Valley Rd., Singapore

Samcax Book Services Ltd., Queensway, P.O. Box 2720, Nairobi, Kenya

First edition 1965

Set in 10 on 12 pt Times
and Printed in Great Britain by
Blackie & Son Ltd., Bishopbriggs, Glasgow

THE CLINICAL PSYCHIATRY
OF LATE LIFE

CONTENTS

FOREWORD

ODD though it may seem, this book was written primarily to satisfy its author's needs. Over more than ten years, one of my main tasks has been to develop a department for patients over the age of 60 at the Bethlem Royal Hospital with out-patient clinics at the Maudsley Hospital. With an annual admission rate of some 130 elderly patients belonging to all diagnostic categories, it has been possible to afford experience with geriatric problems to a large proportion of trainees in psychiatry, holding junior posts or clinical assistantships at this Joint Post-graduate Teaching Hospital. I have found these young colleagues to be a stimulating and highly critical group, and have felt an increasing need to clarify my own experiences and ideas, as well as to bring myself up to date on the subject of ageing as far as it is related to psychiatry. To me, the best way of obtaining a clearer grasp of a subject is through writing: hence this book.

Therefore, my thanks are due first of all to the many junior psychiatrists who have helped me in the treatment of our patients, and to senior and junior members of the Bethlem nursing and occupational therapy staffs. During most of the last ten years, Lady Archibald had been the Psychiatric Social Worker of the geriatric unit, and I am also grateful to her for reading part of the typescript. Dr. J. A. N. Corsellis gave valuable neuropathological advice, and kindly supplied the photographs illustrating various brain changes; thanks are also due to Dr. R. D. Hoare for permission to reproduce X-ray photographs. Finally, I would like to express my gratitude to Dr. W. O. McCormick for his careful and critical reading of the draft manuscript, and for his many constructive suggestions.

FELIX POST

CHAPTER I

HEALTHY AGEING

A STUDY of psychological disturbances of late life ought to be based on a thorough understanding of the mental and physical ageing of healthy persons. Unfortunately, this desirable demand cannot be honoured at the present time for two apparently contradictory reasons—too little is known and too much is written. The physical and psychological aspects of old age have been quite well understood and described by writers and thinkers since antiquity. We shall not here repeat well-quoted passages from the first book of Plato's *Republic* or from Cicero's *De Senectute* (for a recent historical survey see Rosen, 1961). However, Comfort (1961) has reminded us that "the concern of scientists—as against mystics, quacks and therapeutic optimists—with the control of human age processes, if we date it from Metchnikoff and Claude Bernard, is less than a hundred years old; the engagement of science in studying it as an immediately realisable project is less than ten. Gerontology in its modern sense dates from about 1950". Comfort feels that little real progress has so far been made in spite of the veritable torrent of publications, which tends to overwhelm the student trying to obtain a balanced view of normal ageing. A recent classified bibliography of gerontology and geriatrics (Shock, 1963) contains, for the years 1956–61, 18,121 titles! Birren's *Handbook* (1959) consists of 24 chapters, each written by an expert, and the list of references enumerates some 1700 authors. When one tries to apply concepts of ageing to psychiatry, great difficulties arise. These have been lucidly analysed by Aubrey Lewis (1955). All the same, in this first chapter an attempt will be made to present those findings of gerontology which appear to have relevance to the psychiatry of late life. References are given mainly to papers

1

which will guide the reader towards a more searching and thorough study of the various subjects touched upon.

PHYSICAL AGE CHANGES

First a few remarks concerning *physical appearance* in old age. Senile habitus mainly reflects changes in the skin and its appendages, as well as in the locomotor apparatus. The epidermis becomes thin in old age; sweat and sebum glands atrophy; there is diminution of subcutaneous fat, and degeneration of elastic and collagen fibres in connective tissue. There results the dry, thin and wrinkled skin of old people. Hair turns white and becomes more sparse; nails are thickened, rough and brittle. Bones tend to become decalcified, fragile and bent, the spine becoming kyphotic with wedging of vertebrae. Muscle atrophies; gait and other movements, including those of facial expression, are slowed. More severe motility disorders, such as rigidities and tremors, are caused by central nervous system changes which border on the pathological.

Turning from appearances to *functioning*, one finds that a number of physical characteristics do not, at any rate under basal conditions, change with age; the resting level of blood sugar, acid-base equilibrium, the volume of blood and its osmotic pressure, may be given as examples. Many more functions decline: cardiac output, by 30 per cent between the ages of 20 and 90, with peripheral resistance to the flow of blood increasing. Blood-flow through the kidney decreases by 50 per cent. Basal metabolic rate and the oxygen consumption of the body as a whole decrease from the third decade of life onwards. Other functions decline only slightly (e.g. the velocity of neural transmission only by 10 per cent); or only for a time (e.g. the range of accommodation of the eyes rapidly declines between the ages of 20 and 50, but then remains practically unchanged). It must be stressed that all these declines show large individual variations; some individuals at 90, to give but one example, have as good a renal function as the average 50-year-old.

Much more important than any functional decline of various organs with ageing is *decrease of general adaptability*. Some organs are known to decline during foetal life and childhood (e.g. the thymus gland), but this subserves the general trend towards increasing adaptation of the organism as a whole. Here, by "adaptation", is meant the general capacity of organisms to live under continually changing conditions, and ageing has sometimes been defined as decrease in this adaptability. Thus, ageing organisms show less resilience following injury. Stresses produce a greater physiological displacement than in younger subjects, and this takes longer to recover; in a young person the shift in acid-base equilibrium produced by 10 g of sodium carbonate takes 8 hours to recover; in a person of 70 the resting value may not be restored for between 48 and 72 hours. (A guide towards more detailed information will be found in papers by Verzár, 1957, and Himwich, 1962.)

All decreases of function and of functional adaptability can be explained by two kinds of changes, acting singly or in combination: (1) deterioration in the functional capacity of the cells making up the various organs of the body; (2) decline in number of cells, resulting in the availability of fewer functional units. One of the earliest findings of gerontological histology, with which every medical student becomes familiar, is brown atrophy. Intracellular deposits of pigments like lipofuscin are often regarded as clinker substances, but there is no clear indication that these substances do, in fact, interfere with cell function. A good deal of evidence is, however, accumulating that with ageing individual cells suffer decline of functional capacity (summarised by Shock, 1961).[1] Almost certainly in relation to events in the cell nucleus, to which we shall return presently, enzyme actions decrease with age or become deranged, with consequent defects in intracellular protein synthesis (for summary see Albert, 1960). There follows not only increasing inefficiency of the cell as a functioning unit, but ultimately cell death. In confirmation, there is good evidence for a decrease in number of cells composing many organs of the body. Relatively little affected are organs whose cells are not irreversibly post-mitotic, e.g. the liver; on the other hand, 6 per cent of kidney structure is lost in every decade. Most organs are incapable of regeneration, a fact which is of special importance for neurology and psychiatry in relation to the brain. As the cells of the central nervous system govern endocrine and metabolic activities of the body as a whole, neuronal deterioration and death are thought to play the leading role in senescence.

The considerable difficulties encountered in investigating age

[1] And most recently in a paper to the 6th International Congress of Gerontology, *Intrinsic Factors in Ageing* (to be published).

changes in the human brain on account of the frequency of anatomical alterations due to primary cerebral disorders or general disease, as well as of agonal and post-mortem changes, have been fully discussed by Bondareff (1959). Altogether, anatomical studies of old age have proved disappointing (for a review of the last 300 years, see Zeman, 1962). A certain number of facts have, however, been established. Brain-weight begins to decline slowly after the age of 35; this decrease becomes strikingly more rapid after the age of 70, which is interesting because many investigators date real senescence from this age rather than from 60 or 65. Up to the age of 80 there is an increase in the percentage of water and a corresponding decrease of total solids; after 80 this process is reversed, the brain shrinks and cerebrospinal fluid increases in the enlarging ventricles and the widening spaces between brain and skull (Buerger, quoted by Himwich, 1962). Related to this, dried brain-weight ceases to decrease any further after 70, presumably on account of the accumulation of clinker substances and of the replacement of neurones by glial structures. Accordingly, there has been found on chemical analysis a decrease in total protein, lipid content, nitrogen and phosphorus, but an increase of sulphur lipids and lipofuscins, both probably clinker substances. An increase of desoxyribonucleic acid (DNA) is probably due to proliferation of glia, which is less rich in protein and lipin than the replaced neurones. Loss of nerve cells with increasing age and proliferation of glia have been often reported histologically. Experimental studies also favour loss of neurones as the chief cause of frequently confirmed reduction in oxygen utilisation by the aged brain (see Himwich and Himwich, 1959; Himwich, 1962). This finding, as well as the significance of senile plaques and of neurofibrillary changes, will occupy us again when we come to consider senile dementia (Chapter III).

THEORIES OF AGEING

Before going on from this brief summary of physical changes to a consideration of the psychological aspects of ageing, something should be said about the biological problem. A leading characteristic of life processes is their irreversibility, the fact that they are tied to the passage of time. Biologically speaking, ageing describes the changes which occur in living forms with units of time lived, and thus takes its place among other properties of living matter whose natures are equally unknown. In medical literature and common parlance, ageing is the colloquial term for senescence: increase in years accompanied by decline of bodily functions, sensibilities and energies.

Developing the ideas of earlier biologists like Minot and Weismann, Medawar (1957) has formulated a modern hypothesis of ageing. He reminds us that there are two kinds of senescence: there is senescence which is "comprised of the accumulated sum of the effect of recurrent stress or injury or infection" which is of environmental origin; but there is also "the innate or ingrained senescence which is, in a general sense, developmental or the effect of 'nature' ". Medawar arrives at the following definition of senescence: ". . . that change of the bodily faculties and sensibilities and energies which accompanies ageing, and which renders the individual progressively more likely to die from accidental causes." He makes a further important point when he goes on: "Strictly speaking the word 'accidental' is redundant, for all deaths are in some degree accidental. No death is wholly 'natural'; no one dies *merely* of the burden of the years."

We saw earlier that the physical changes which render organisms progressively more likely to die from innate causes are largely the results of deterioration and death of individual cells, consequent upon changes in the functions of the cell nucleus. These, in turn, are determined by chromosomal molecular structure, and a number of recent approaches to the problem of senescence all point to the leading role of information stored in chromosomal material and of changes affecting it.

First of all, duration of life of members of any species depends not only on rate of metabolism, but is also genetically determined (for summary, see Kallmann, 1961). Longevity potential is sex-linked: in almost all species females live longer than males. Moreover, in Man, and in a number of animals, it has been demonstrated that longevity is an inherited characteristic. A great age is most likely to be reached by the offspring when both parents have been long-lived. The additional finding that long-lived fathers tend to have long-lived daughters, and that the same holds as between mothers and sons, has not been fully confirmed so far. Kallmann's twin studies demonstrated that the differences in duration of life of monozygous twin pairs were half that of the differences found in dizygous twins (monozygous: average difference, 36·9 months; dizygous, same sex,

78·3 months; and dizygous, different sex, 126·6 months). Moreover, age changes in appearance and causes of death tended to be strikingly similar in identical twins. A multifactorial type of inheritance is assumed for life-span potential.

Senescence may be regarded not only as genetically determined, but also as the result of the forces of natural selection (Medawar, 1957). For promoting the survival of the species, the individual female ceases to be effective as soon as her ovaries have emptied, and in fact only Man and domestic animals under his protection tend to survive into the post-productive period of life. Even before this stage has been reached, progressively increasing numbers of any population will have died from a variety of accidental causes, and by reason of their numerical superiority alone, the youngest members make the greatest contribution towards the continuation of the species. Thus, a deleterious gene which manifests its effects early in life will be eliminated speedily through natural selection; a harmful gene manifesting itself later will be bred out more slowly, with the age of manifestation being gradually postponed. Deleterious genes which manifest themselves only during the post-reproductive period of life are not eliminated at all. There is then, towards late life, a considerable accumulation of harmful genes which are no longer eliminated by the process of natural selection.

In addition it has been suggested that harmful genes also arise *de novo* during life by mutation, and that this may be the predominant cause of senescence (summarised by Comfort, 1961). The rate of ageing may thus be regarded as a function of the sum of all mutagenic influences on the body; it is suspected that one of them is ionising radiation of cosmic origin. Mutations are produced by "hits" scored on chromosomes by radiation. These are random events, which remain constant throughout life, and the number of "hits" registered increases with time lived (Szillard, 1959). Burnet (1959) has suggested ageing might be essentially the integration of mutational damage to somatic cells; their effect on the antibody functioning of cells of the reticulo-endothelial system and the subsequent increase of auto-immune reactions with rising age may well be one of the mechanisms underlying the infirmities and loss of vigour in ageing (Comfort, 1961).

It thus seems reasonable to explain the occurrence of senescence as due to an accumulation of harmful genes, from a variety of causes, towards the time when the female ceases to contribute to the continuation of the species. To return to Medawar's definition of senescence, both the female at this time and her male partner are, on account of this accumulation of deleterious genes, "progressively more likely to die from accidental causes". Verzár (1957) has drawn a graphic picture of ageing Primitive Man: by the age of 50, when ovulation has ceased in the female, her (and her male companion's) capacity to accommodate visually has reached its end. They will still be able to recognise their neighbours in the cave, but will not notice until it is too late their enemies in the jungle. This picture is, of course, a trifle overdrawn in that many people over 50 retain sufficient visual acuity to survive even under primitive conditions; other results of senescence would, however, make their continued existence increasingly unlikely. Verzár goes on to point out that after reaching the end of the reproductive period of life, both men and women are from a narrowly biological point of view superfluous for the maintenance of the race. We may go further and suggest that, by removing biologically useless individuals, senescence emerges in animals as a powerful agent which ensures the survival of the species; a strain encumbered by increasing numbers of individuals who no longer contribute to its proliferation would eventually succumb in the struggle for existence, with other species favoured by the occurrence of senescence and of "natural" death.

Man stands out in the animal kingdom by reason of his capacity to store and elaborate life experiences mentally, and to transfer them by speech to other members of his species. In a wider sense than the merely biological one, he remains useful to his race after his reproductive role is over. We shall resist the temptation of calling on Anthropology and History to pursue the suggestion that those human races have been most successful in surviving who have produced the best senates. Instead, we shall turn to a discussion of the senescence of the mind.

THE AGEING MIND

It will be convenient as well as meaningful to deal with this subject under three sub-headings: (1) changes in cognitive functions, i.e. in intellectual, as well as in sensorimotor performance; (2) changes with age in the emotional and motivational aspects of personality; (3) changes in relationships with others, i.e. in social functioning.

INTELLECTUAL PERFORMANCE

If we define intelligence quite naïvely as those aspects of behaviour which are measurable by intelligence tests—then there is no doubt of its deterioration with advancing years. Test performance reaches its peak during the second or third decade of life, and from then on shows progressive decline. However, the age of optimum performance and the rate and extent of decline vary with the ability measured. In addition, Wechsler (1961) points out that it is debatable whether intelligence tests measure all that is generally called intelligence, and suggests that intelligence ought to be defined differently at different ages: "At younger ages, definitions of intelligence are likely to emphasise mental alertness, ability to learn and capacity to see new relationships. In older ages one is more concerned with what is broadly covered by the terms wisdom and sagacity, where by sagacity one means the ability to deal with life's situations in terms of past experience." On analysis, the standardisation data of the Wechsler Adult Intelligence Scale showed no decline up to the age of 64 in general intelligence (a component which was probably identical with Spearman's factor g). With rising age there was an increase in the number of words recognised and of factual items correctly given on an information test. However, ageing was found to make considerable inroads on mental ability in test situations calling for an analysis of percepto-spatial relations (Birren, 1961). At a higher age, abstract reasoning (Jones, 1957) and the ability to adopt an abstract attitude in sorting tests (Hopkins and Post, 1955) were found to become increasingly impaired.

It is common knowledge that memory declines with rising age, and there is a general observation (Ribot's law) that material acquired early in life is retained longest. What we loosely call "memory" is in fact a highly complex process involving a number of functions, all of which have attracted much research. Two of them have special relevance to the problems of old people: the first, short-term memory, will occupy us a little later; the other, which is the ability to reproduce recently acquired information, i.e. learning ability, declines severely with increasing age. This occurs also in animals (in maze-learning by rats, Verzár-McDougal, 1957). Gilbert (1941) demonstrated that age-decline in learning ability differed with the type of task. Comparing subjects aged 20–29 with subjects aged 60–69, she found that there was only a 12 per cent loss in auditory memory-span for digits. For repeating sentences the loss was 21 per cent, for whole paragraphs 40 per cent and for the retention of word pairs 55 per cent. Kral (1962) has pointed out the differences which exist between the memory difficulties of healthy old people and those associated with senile dementia, and other evidence suggesting that the decline of all intellectual functioning with age is not only less severe, but also much more orderly than that seen in dementing illnesses, will be presented in Chapter III.

SENSORIMOTOR PERFORMANCE

Slowness is a well-recognised characteristic of old age. It presents an increasing handicap of the ageing worker in industry, and at a higher age it may cause difficulties in general adjustment. This subject has been lucidly reviewed for a medical audience by Welford (1962). It used to be thought that slowing of sensorimotor activities was due to changes in the receptor and effector organs; that older people comprehended more slowly because their visual and auditory receptor mechanisms were defective, and that they acted more slowly because their motor mechanisms, especially co-ordination, had deteriorated. No doubt, many old people become less skilled on account of sensory handicaps and neuromuscular disorders, but experimental work has recently demonstrated that the main cause of slowing lies in the central mechanisms of perceiving signals and of shaping actions in response to them.

In applying information-theory to brain function, we may picture neurone cells as continually generating impulses, and assume that this random neural activity creates continuous "neural noise". This forms the background to the transmission of signals within the central nervous system, which thus have to continue for some time before they are successfully distinguished from the background noise, and before they are picked up by receiving neurones. Transmission of impulses will be slowed under two conditions: (1) when the signals are weakened, and (2) when the background neural noise from which they have to be differentiated is increased. Loss of available neurones, and impairment of their function, which we saw occurred in ageing, will weaken the strength of signals generated by cell assemblies. There is also a good deal of evidence (which Welford cites) that neural noise increases in the ageing brain. A combination of both these factors may well form the neurophysiological basis of sensori-motor slowing in ageing.

The decline of *short-term retention* with age may also be explained by applying information-theory to cerebral physiology. We noted earlier that the number of digits which can be repeated back immediately is little affected by ageing. Old people perform well on the digit-span test, but tend to fall down badly as soon as another activity is interposed between perception and repetition. It has been postulated that short-term memory is stored in memory traces, which are now thought to be self-exciting neural circuits. These circuits eventually tend to run down or become broken up by the surrounding neural noise. We may thus picture the memory traces of older persons to be weaker on account of the decreased functional capacity and available number of brain cells, and also to be more quickly extinguished by the louder neural noise.

Impaired short-term retention is probably a factor in poor memory for recent experiences (see also Caird and Inglis, 1961). It presents an obvious handicap to learning new material and new skills, especially when instructions have to be carried in the head as the task proceeds. Repetition of instructions and the provision of additional cues may help to raise the level of performance. If tasks are speeded (in industry or in the laboratory) the effects of slowing make themselves felt, and an old person tends to become overloaded. As long as the older worker is allowed to take his time, no loss of skill occurs; otherwise he may omit some action, sacrifice accuracy for speed, or he may simplify actions by restricting himself to certain aspects of his task. Welford suggests that this tendency may lie at the bottom of the narrowing of interests and restriction of activities so often seen in the elderly. The only area in which old age surpasses youth is the increase of knowledge and experience; but the very possession of this wealth of information may make appropriate decisions more difficult and lead to vacillating behaviour. Older people have learnt to recognise ways in which groups of objects and sequences of events hang together. This makes the handling of situations easier, but the excessive use by elderly people of these patterns of thought and action leads to yet another of their characteristics, namely increased rigidity.

In summary, we may point out that the organisation of mental abilities alters with age in a way which is well suited to the changing demands presented by successive life periods. The ability to learn new skills and new facts is of foremost importance in the young; without it a young animal could not learn to survive outside the nest, and the young person could not reach an independent position in life. Later on, when most of the things which can be learnt have been learnt, the ability to organise mental experience and to economise effort becomes more important. At the lowest level of human endeavour, older people often do their work more neatly and more reliably than younger workers; at the highest level, older persons are able to draw on their store of experience and knowledge, recognise significant patterns, and make decisions which take into consideration many factors and imponderables. Mathematicians, historians, legal authorities and statesmen, for all these reasons, usually attain their highest level of achievement late in life. By contrast, scientists, creative artists in every field, poets and writers tend to produce their best work before the age of 40; their creations demand experiencing and integrating new facts, fresh impressions or warm feelings.

EMOTIONAL AGEING

We saw just now that cognitive age changes may lie at the bottom of some personality characteristics of elderly people. Precise measurements are not possible in the area of emotion and motivation, and researchers have to rely on the use of various questionnaires, inventories and projection tests administered to members of different age groups. Longitudinal, biographical studies of personality change tend to have been made only in outstanding and thus unrepresentative people. The literature on emotional ageing is not only large, but often contradictory: to give but one example, some studies suggest that religious interests increase with rising age, while others deny this. For those seeking detailed information, Birren's *Handbook* (1959) contains summary articles on drives, expectancies and emotions, on personality theory and ageing, and on ageing and life adjustment. This last subject will be dealt with in a later section of the present chapter; here, we shall give an outline of personality developments with ageing which have special relevance to psychiatry. Most themes will be taken up again in the chapter (VI) concerned with personality disorders.

In healthy people, adult personality structure tends to remain remarkably stable throughout life; people grow old, as they have lived. Only minor shifts of orientation may be discerned. Presumably in relation to their greater need and capacity to learn, younger persons tend to be strongly orientated towards the outside world. With increasing age there is a shift from extroversion to introversion. People, as they grow older, tend to turn inwardly, and this trend goes a long way to explain many frequently attested differences between the young and the old. Older people are more family centred; they prefer activities which are not only less strenuous, but which can be pursued alone or in company with only one person. With an increasing disinclination to learning, elderly people often show a pronounced tendency to resist changing their beliefs and opinions. However, individual variations are considerable, and the stereotype of a rigid conservatism of the aged is very much exaggerated. Around the age of 40, transitory anxieties may arise in relation to dissatisfactions with jobs, careers and marriages. From the sixth decade onwards there is an increasing tendency towards a worried outlook and emotional over-reaction to stress, which may diminish after the age of 70 has been reached. Undue interests in, and concerns over, bodily functions are well-known features of late middle life, which once again indicate increasing tendencies towards introversion with rising age. By contrast, many personality features of younger people tend to reflect a need to control drives and impulses which threaten to impinge unduly on the outside world, especially on other persons and on society.

Of these outwardly directed drives, the sexual is probably the most powerful one, which is often held to be basic to aggressive and acquisitive trends. *Changes in sexual function* are strikingly associated with ageing, and strength and orientation of sexual libido are, in turn, related to many other personality features. Senescent personality changes, such as increased preoccupation with the body (especially with bowel function), rigidity, tendency to patterned and stereotyped behaviour, and anxious parsimoniousness, may all be explained in psychoanalytical terms as due to a shift from genital to anal libidinal orientation. All available evidence certainly points to a marked decrease with increasing age of genital sexuality, which (in males) reaches its greatest intensity in the late teens. Throughout adult life, male sexuality follows a linear decline; change of partner may for a time cause an increase of coital frequency, but the previous pattern of steady decline soon becomes re-established (Kinsey *et al.*, 1948). Far less is known of the effects of ageing on the psychological aspects of female sexuality, though Kinsey and his colleagues (1953) thought that, allowing for cultural and social restrictions, libidinal changes were slight up to the period of old age. Until recently little was known concerning the sexuality of old people, except that it was well preserved in some; the mistress of the aged Louis XIV used to complain of the excessive demands made on her! Newman and Nichols (1960) demonstrated that habit was perhaps the strongest factor leading to continued sexual activity. Only a few widowed or divorced voluntary informants aged 60–93 admitted to still having sexual intercourse; some complained of frustration, but the desire was rarely strong enough to lead to extramarital relations (in only 7 per cent). Between the ages of 60 and 75 there was no decline in the proportion of married men and women who enjoyed regular inter-course; around 60 per cent remained sexually active. This proportion diminished rapidly after the age of 75, with an overall 25 per cent remaining sexually active. Chronic ill health was the most frequently given cause for discontinuing marital relations. Old people who remained sexually potent uniformly rated themselves as having been strongly or moderately strongly sexed when young; old people who described themselves as without sexual feelings claimed that their interest had never been strong. In most old people, libido and potency tend to diminish concomitantly; this is, unfortunately, not the case in those exhibiting sexual behaviour disorders (see Chapter VI).

Awareness of the increasing likelihood of death might be thought to affect the emotional and motivational aspects of ageing personalities. Certainly there is with increasing age a tendency for people to feel that time (psychological time) is running out ever more quickly. This frequently reported phenomenon has never been satisfactorily explained. An interesting mathematical theory has been worked out by Mitchell (1957), according to which the duration of an interval in psychological time is subjectively measured by comparison with the total apparent duration of life up to a specific reference date; the longer the duration of life (i.e. the larger the denominator), the shorter will appear the subjective duration of a recent period. Studies of attitudes towards death have produced variable and contradictory results; some suggest that fear of death is a problem of adolescence, others that it is specially related to old age. Whether or not religious attitudes correlate with death attitudes forms another controversial subject. At the conclusion of a symposium on death attitudes, Munnichs (1961) pointed out that results depended very much on the research instruments (interviews, questionnaires, or projective techniques) used. All that emerged clearly was: "Attitude toward death, in so far as this attitude is *fear* of death, makes its appearance whenever we deal with persons who are not mentally healthy." Death certainly is one of the main (not necessarily fully conscious) preoccupations of affectively or neurotically ill old people. Even among dements, the concept of death retains realistic significance (Abraham, 1962). Investigating a group of general hospital patients with fatal illnesses, Hinton (1963) found that some 40 per cent came to realise that death was either probable or certain. This was no more frequently the case in older than in younger patients. Anxiety and depression were more often seen in patients who admitted that they were aware of the proximity of death; affective changes were a little more common in younger patients facing death (Hinton, personal communication). Exton-Smith (1961) reported that a similar proportion of mentally clear elderly people (42 per cent) realised during their terminal illness that they were going to die soon; but only a handful seemed restless and anxious, largely on account of distressing physical conditions. There are, then, some definite pointers towards a calmer acceptance of death by older people.

This attitude, the waning of sexual drives, the decline of outwardly directed tendencies, and the maintained ability to utilise to best advantage intellectual capital rather than to acquire new information —all these may be interpreted as changes in personality structure, which serve persons entering old age to advantage. During the post-reproductive period, natural selection can be invoked no longer to explain the occurrence of these (from the point of view of adaptation) favourable characteristics. However, Birren (1960) has suggested that these orderly and biologically useful changes occurring during the post-reproductive period may be related as "counterparts" to earlier characteristics, which *are* subject to the pressures of natural selection. He quotes results of genetic animal experiments in longevity, which are in keeping with his counterpart theory of ageing. We may add that vigorous and intelligent people tend to stand up better to the effects of senescence than poorly endowed persons, and that centenarians have almost always been exceptionally well adjusted throughout life.

SOCIAL ASPECTS OF AGEING

In the course of the preceding discussion, my own orientation towards the problem of ageing will have become clear. I have attempted to show that, from the biological–evolutional point of view, death was necessary, but that as far as Man was concerned, the senescent individual continued to make, by reason of his mental qualities, important contributions to the survival of his species. We went on to discover that later personality developments led to a re-patterning of functions, which thus became particularly well suited to the lives of men and women during the post-reproductive period. This approach presents a reaction against earlier scientific research and theorising in ageing which has done "little more than reflect and reinforce the current negative stereotype about the ageing process, especially the all too prevalent concept of deterioration" (Arnhoff, 1961).

We shall not follow the common practice of drawing attention to the relative increase of the elderly in the population of civilised countries and the consequent health problems (for the most recent summary see Wolff, 1963). Eventually, a new age structure based on a lower birth rate and shaped by a greater survival rate will become established in these populations, and the appropriate social policies will be worked out. At present large sections of the elderly suffer hardships, but to judge from surveys in town and country (e.g. Sheldon, 1948; Miller, 1963), the great majority do not break down mentally under the considerable stresses they have to bear. Except during severe or terminal illness, institutional care becomes necessary mainly in those who on account of great age have outlived their families and friends (a very small minority), and to some extent in old people who have become isolated through blows of misfortune, e.g. having been widowed and left with no or few children. In a considerable proportion of old people requiring institutional care, this need arises because they have become socially isolated as an inevitable aftermath of lifelong neurotic and other personality difficulties. Adequate care of elderly persons in distress, from whatever cause, is a matter for public conscience; medical workers should most certainly draw the attention of the community to these problems, but should be careful not to overstate their case.

Criticisms of the attitude of the modern family to its aged members are a case in point. Investigations, such as those carried out by Townsend (1957) in a working-class district, and by Willmott and Young (1960) in a residential suburb, have shown that, in spite of economic difficulties, the status of elderly people in the modern family remains on the whole satisfactory, with elderly women being in an especially favourable position on account of their close relationship with daughters and granddaughters. Retirement is another social problem which has given rise to many indignant protests. It is frequently cited (most recently by Wolff, 1963) as the commonest precipitating cause of psychological breakdown in the elderly, but sociological studies (summarised by Welford, 1958) ascertained that retirement turned out to be compulsory in only 25 per cent of men; physical and psychological ill health (most of it vague) were far more common causes of failure to continue in employment. Anticipation of compulsory retirement often caused much dread and anxiety (Lorge and Tuckman, 1953), but after it had taken place there tended to be a marked increase of adjustment and satisfaction (Thompson and Suchman, 1958). Most healthy and well-adjusted men retired gradually, in that they continued in part-time work (Richardson, 1956).

Very much in line with the optimistic views adopted here are the contributions by Cumming and Henry (1961). They pointed out that many previous sociological investigations suffered from a tendency of estimating the characteristics of old people in terms of the sociologist's own value system. As these researchers were mostly young, and as they tended to belong socially to the middle classes, it was not surprising that they reported lowered morale in elderly people on the basis of negative responses to questions like "Do you still feel useful to others?" They appeared to make the latent assumption that successful ageing consisted in being as much like a middle-aged person as possible. There are, it must be admitted, many studies which have quite objectively demonstrated positive correlations between the emotional condition of old people and the number of roles they continued to play. They have all tended to show that subjects were reported by themselves and by their friends as happiest whenever they remained occupied, participant and in contact with many other persons. On the other hand, old people of this kind were, statistically speaking, abnormal. In one study (Albrecht, 1951), they accounted for only 35 per cent; lessening of interests, of activities and of interpersonal contacts were much more frequently seen. Cumming and Henry (1961) followed a group of elderly people over a number of years, and their findings were in keeping with a Disengagement Theory of Ageing. With rising age they found steady diminution of interaction with other people. Contacts with intimates did not diminish (except on account of death or moving away). Disengagement did also occur from kin, but this shift was not so much in the amount of interaction as in the quality of the relationship. There was a move from love-seeking to dependency; very old people finally took little interest in people other than with reference to their own needs—very much like children. They also tended to be much more satisfied and to accept the proximity of death better than slightly younger subjects. As people grew older they developed greater narrowness and rigidity of outlook, which was increasingly uninfluenced by general views and norms. Old men especially tended to get more and more satisfaction from dwelling on memories of past successes and achievements, and from creating a self-image of the wise old man who can indulge in sweeping statements without fear of criticism from others. Mainly for men, but also for an increasing number of women, retirement may be regarded as an enforced and sudden form of disengagement. It spells not only loss of status, but also loss of contact with many persons outside the family. Most men in Cumming and Henry's study were able to reduce these stresses by taking part-time jobs or by engaging in activities (hobbies and interests) which were only remotely related to their past jobs. However, these were temporary expedients, which were soon given up, but which served the purpose of making the disengagement process a more gradual one.

Widowing is an event which is much more devastating than retirement. In this respect, men are in an even more unfortunate position than women, who are eventually able to re-attach themselves to other persons, especially to other widows. These new relationships tended (according to Cumming and Henry) to be less demanding than the former ones, and were in line with the process of disengagement. The disengaged woman might even become more frivolous, with a desire to gallivant around, a passion for coach tours, etc. In many cases this behaviour might, however, be a defence against a deeper sense of unhappiness.

Unfortunately, all these positive results of disengagement with ageing tend to be much modified by poverty, ill health and previous personality difficulties. Another study (Reichard *et al.*, 1962) reported that men who had always been relatively free of neurotic conflicts, and who had found satisfaction in activities and personal relationships, were able to disengage without regrets for the past or sense of loss in the present. Another type ("rocking-chair men") had always been generally passive, and welcomed the opportunity to be free of responsibility. They had adopted passive attitudes in life, had been under-aggressive, but at the same time self-indulgent, especially as regards eating and drinking. "Armoured" men were unable to disengage completely. They could not face passivity or helplessness in old age, and appeared to ward off anxiety and dread of physical decline by keeping active. Unsatisfactory disengagement tended to occur in men who always had a hostile attitude towards the world, which they regarded as a jungle. They often became seclusive with age, harboured almost grandiose ideas about their own value and would not occupy themselves. In others, lifelong inferiority feelings led to a sense of disappointment, self-hatred and a depressive outlook.

CONCLUDING REMARKS

Looked at from the standpoint of earlier adult life, old age is a period of decline. When assessed in relation to the evolution and preservation of the human species, the changes occurring in late life can be shown to be conducive to optimal adaptation. What are losses in the eyes of younger persons, such as decline of sexual libido, of interest in other people, of desire to learn, of ability to remember what happened yesterday—none of these changes are causes of subjective dissatisfaction and unhappiness in most old people.

Unfortunately, with increasing age men and women are more and more exposed to influences, which disturb the gradual and orderly process of withdrawal and disengagement characteristic of ideal old age. Many physical illnesses used to cut off the life of elderly people abruptly without affecting adjustment. Gone are the days when pneumonia was called "the old man's friend", and frequently recurring or chronically disabling illnesses tend to lead to a medicated, but not often enjoyable, extended existence. Increasing loneliness and isolation are other results of modern conditions of life, but their importance has probably been exaggerated. The fact that the duration of life has been prolonged for many people with personality weaknesses and with deleterious genes of late manifestation, is probably the main factor which is responsible for the heavy incidence of psychiatric disorders in old age.

Between the ages of 25 and 75 there is a sixfold increase of the likelihood of being admitted to a mental hospital. Norris (1959) gave the following well-founded estimates: out of every 1000 boys born in London, 8 will be admitted for schizophrenia, 8 for manic-depressive (including involutional) psychoses and 21 for one of the psychoses of old age, at least once during their lifetime. For 1000 girls she gives the following figures: 10 for schizophrenia, 14 for affective psychoses and 28 for old age psychoses. We shall see that affective disorders mostly manifest themselves for the first time after the age of 55, and this, together with the fact that many more elderly persons are psychiatrically affected than are ever admitted to hospital, drives home the realisation that psychological illnesses are very largely disorders of the elderly. There is then no need to give further reasons why every doctor should acquire a working knowledge of the clinical psychiatry of late life.

CHAPTER II

PSYCHIATRIC SYNDROMES AND THEIR DIFFERENTIATION

PSYCHIATRIC DIAGNOSIS IN ELDERLY PATIENTS

Psychiatric illnesses may manifest themselves by physical symptoms and signs like constipation, loss of weight, a dry mouth, furred tongue, increased sweating, changes in heart rate and blood pressure, increased muscle tone, tremors or cataplexy. Disorders of awareness, mood, perception, thinking, or thought content are always present and, as a rule, more prominent. These physiological and psychological symptoms point to disorders of the central nervous and neuro-endocrine systems. In the so-called organic mental states, impairment of awareness and cognitive function is associated with defects or pathological changes in the brain, and usually there are also some positive neurological findings. In some organic psychoses causation is known, e.g. syphilis or coal-gas poisoning; in others, pathological findings permit of classification, e.g. vascular or parenchymal degeneration—but the underlying causes of these pathological changes are unknown. When we come to disorders of behaviour, thinking and experiencing not associated with demonstrable brain changes, we are forced to fall back on multiple causation, assuming an interplay of poorly defined constructs such as inherited and acquired constitution, life situations and stresses. Furthermore, functional mental disorders can only be classified descriptively according to their symptomatology. Different kinds of symptoms tend to cluster together forming syndromes, to which names have been given, e.g. a saddened mood tends to go together with mental slowing, with self-reproachful ideation and suicidal behaviour (melancholia); or anxious and worrying people may at times exhibit

20

physical symptoms of anxiety with irrational fears and senseless repetitions of thoughts or actions (phobic-obsessive states). However, many patients tend to suffer from symptoms belonging to several clusters, and their illnesses are then called atypical. It is not surprising that a typical course or response to treatment is seen far less commonly in psychiatric disorders than in cases of fractured femur, of pneumococcal lobar pneumonia or of general paralysis of the insane (basically a physical disorder).

There is no need to labour the point any further; psychiatric diagnoses have to be made within a framework of incomplete knowledge and provisional nosological classifications, which are much influenced by the school of thought to which individual psychiatrists belong, and by the teachings prevalent in the country where they work. On the other hand, diagnosing psychiatric patients does lead to an appreciation of some of the things that have gone wrong, and to ways of managing and treating patients successfully, in a fair proportion of patients. Careful examination and assessment followed by diagnostic evaluation are not, therefore, futile or academic exercises.

In the elderly the situation is even more complex. Symptoms tend to suggest the presence of more than one psychiatric disorder, and in addition patients often suffer from one or more physical illnesses or disabilities. It is not, however, sufficient to make a multidimensional diagnosis, as this may lead to an attitude of therapeutic nihilism or to trial and error procedures, with no single treatment being given sufficiently intensively or over a long enough period. The clinician should endeavour to deepen his diagnostic understanding of the patient by unravelling the essential from the less essential in terms of causal relationships, likely response to treatment and long-term management.

Let us take the hypothetical case of a man who is 72 years old and who has been referred on account of restlessness and aggressive behaviour. He is found to be impaired in memory and to be to some extent disorientated; in addition he believes that his money has gone, and he blames himself for some alleged past dishonesty. Physically, he has a cough and moist sounds in his chest, but no fever. Assessment of this patient should proceed along the following lines:

Physical state: With a fuller history, physical examination and investigations it will be possible to determine which of the three most likely conditions is present: chronic bronchitis, broncho-pneumonia (frequently non-febrile in the aged!) or congestive heart failure. Chronic bronchitis is probably a coincidental finding, but broncho-pneumonia or cardiac failure are much more likely precipitants of mental symptoms, on account of toxaemia or anoxia.

The cognitive defect may be due to cerebral pathological changes. Where the defect arose acutely, without any history of gradual decline, we are most likely dealing with an *acute confusional state* (acute brain syndrome, senile delirium). This diagnosis is made more likely if there is also a physical illness producing toxaemia or anoxia.

On the other hand, a history of intellectual and personality decline over many months or, more often, years, suggests that the basic disorder is a *chronic confusional state* (chronic brain syndrome), and at this age *senile dementia* or *arteriosclerotic dementia* are the commonest more specific diagnoses.

In the presence of toxic or anoxic factors of recent origin, we may be dealing with a *secondary* and often *terminal confusional state* complicating one of the dementias of old age.

Ideas of guilt and poverty may be due to personality features colouring the psychological disturbance produced by the cerebral disorder, but, especially when features of the organic psychosyndrome are mild, the presence of an *affective illness* must be considered. Aggressive and hostile behaviour with restlessness may be due to *manic* components, but *melancholia* in one of its many varieties is a much more likely diagnosis in our hypothetical case.

In the presence of aggressive behaviour and a hostile attitude, exploration may reveal paranoid attitudes, beliefs or experiences. Again, these may be due to personality features modifying the symptomatology of an organic psychosis, or they may point to the diagnosis of a *persecutory syndrome* (late paraphrenia, schizophrenia).

Unravelling the complex features of our hypothetical (but by no means unusual) case has led us to set out the diagnostic classification adopted in this book, which is completed by adding *psychoneuroses* and *personality disorders* as seen in elderly people. In subsequent chapters we shall describe more fully these different syndromes, the ways in which they tend to be associated with one another and the methods of treating them. However, in diagnosing patients a variety of techniques are used. Many are applicable in all types of disorder, and these will be discussed now.

TECHNIQUES OF CLINICAL ASSESSMENT

Readers of this book are assumed to have practical experience of neuropsychiatric case taking, a subject which has been described very fully and recently by R. S. Allison in his book *The Senile Brain* (1962). However, experience has taught me that there are a number of aspects of history-taking and mental examination which are not fully understood by doctors unfamiliar with disturbed elderly patients, and I shall also deal in this chapter with the ways of interpreting the results of some ancillary procedures such as psychological testing, electro- and pneumoencephalography.

HISTORY-TAKING

Disordered behaviour, talk, mood, thinking, imagining and experiencing, as well as physical abnormalities, variously contribute to the clinical pictures presented by psychiatric patients. In the preceding section we sought to demonstrate that these features could be the result of a number of different conditions. In many instances of common psychiatric illnesses an experienced observer will be able to make a correct diagnosis by recognising familiar combinations of signs and symptoms. Where patients have been living alone and in little contact with other people, decisions about treatment and management may have to be made, *faute de mieux*, on the basis of their mental and physical state as well as that of their homes, their bodies and their clothing. In many instances a complete and reliable assessment is possible only when we are able to find out how long ago a disorder had first been noticed, the sequence in which various symptoms and disabilities had appeared and the speed with which they have increased. Furthermore, the repertoire of psychological symptomatology is limited, and similar clinical pictures (in analogy with the "final common path" of neurology) may be due to a variety of pathological happenings. Finally, by adding the longitudinal view of the history to the cross-section obtained through examining the patient, we may be able to foresee the developments which are likely to occur unless treatment results in a significant change.

Where patients come for consultation with mild, subjective complaints, it is often sufficient, and indeed instructive, to learn from them how they believe their difficulties have arisen. Present symptoms

2   CPLL

and attitudes, as well as a subjective account of their previous life experience, may be illuminating, and may point to fruitful lines of treatment. Sooner or later the psychiatrist will try to get patients to accept that their difficulties can be fully understood and satisfactorily dealt with only in relation to the attitudes and feelings of people close to them. Contact with their friends may correct one's view of the patients' problems, and lead one to modify their treatment.

The majority of elderly patients are seriously ill by the time they are referred for specialist advice on account of psychological problems. Though it is good practice, even in the most disturbed patients, to foster the idea that they have come to get help by encouraging them to give a personal account of their difficulties, the results may in fact be grossly misleading. Histories obtained from dementing, persecuted or depressed patients are, after all, part of their mental states, reflecting their thought content and preoccupations. As a rule, better contact can be established with patients of this type after a preliminary history has been taken from the person accompanying them. In many instances the friends of elderly patients will themselves be senile in mentality and outlook, and, to an even greater extent than in the case of younger patients, it will not be sufficient merely to listen to the informants' stories. These may be limited to a recital of reputed causes of the patient's disorders or to the informants' own difficulties—in themselves important pieces of information. It is good practice to listen for a few minutes in order to establish good contact, but then a systematic inquiry will have to follow.

In psychiatry, as in other branches of medicine, a good history may yield many more significant leads towards a correct diagnosis than some ancillary investigations. It is instructive to obtain full knowledge of the patient's background, i.e. his heredity, childhood, work record, sexual and marital experiences. By contrast, descriptions of previous personality traits, following some schedule or other, tend to conceal more than they reveal, and different informants frequently give conflicting accounts. A full description of the symptoms observed during previous episodes of ill health, as well as of the course of earlier disorders, may help to explain and evaluate the significance of present clinical features. In the process of eliciting from his friends the patient's recent symptoms and the sequence in which they appeared, various diagnostic pointers will have begun to emerge.

Their significance, as well as the ways in which they may be turned to best use, are not always appreciated, and merit fuller discussion.

(1) *Duration and mode of onset.* Almost all psychiatric illnesses tend to be irreversible, or only partly reversible, when symptoms have been continuously present for more than two or three years. Duration of illness is also a valuable diagnostic indicator; mental decline and other symptoms due to the dementias of old age usually progress over long periods before they are noticed (except in retrospect) by relatives and friends, and before patients are finally referred by their family doctors for specialist's advice. A short history of intellectual difficulties is much more suggestive of rapidly progressive cerebral disorders, such as some cerebrovascular processes, intoxications, syphilitic inflammations or neoplasms. However, relatives often date first symptoms from a recent, emotionally significant event, such as the death of a spouse or loss of home, and probably the patient's condition had worsened considerably after one of these losses of social support. But on closer and more searching inquiry, the patient's friends are likely to recall events and observations pointing to a decline of abilities for some time before the traumatic event. Some depressive illnesses in middle-aged and elderly people with personality difficulties also run a long and insidiously worsening course, but usually there is a history of well-marked fluctuations as well.

It is important to discover the exact nature of the very first symptoms, even though at the time they had been ignored or accepted as "due to his age" by the family. Most chronic organic psychoses begin with memory difficulties (inability to recall the names of people, missing appointments, repeated requests for information, repetitive relating of recent and remote experiences), episodes of disorientation (especially at night), or failure to recognise persons. More subtle changes of personality and character are hardly ever noticed by the average family, and ill-defined anxiety and depressive symptoms are uncommon precursors of dementia. By contrast, forgetfulness or muddledness in carrying out simple household tasks may be symptoms of a depressive illness, but in this case the history tends to be a short one, and depressive symptoms are obvious by the time the patient is seen.

(2) *Reasons for referral.* These are usually self-evident in cases of recent onset. Where there is a long history of ill health, referral is often precipitated by confusional episodes (due to intercurrent

physical disease) in the course of a dementing process, or by social reasons, such as the moving away or ill health of relatives, making continued home care difficult. In long-standing depressions advice may be sought because the patient has made a suicidal attempt or gesture. By the time the patient is seen, relatives may try to conceal this, and specific inquiries may have to be made. Quite apart from diagnostic considerations, it is essential to discover the true reason for which a patient is referred for specialist's advice after a long period of mental invalidism. Neither the family doctor nor the relatives are likely to say outright: "We have called you in because this situation has become unbearable, and we want you to relieve us from this burden." And yet this is the case in many consultations, and the family atmosphere may have grown so tense that temporary admission to hospital may be a social, if not clinical, necessity. We shall discuss the management of such situations in the last chapter. Domiciliary consultation may not be the best setting in which to make an exact clinical diagnosis, but it is almost indispensable whenever it is equally or even more important to arrive at a social diagnosis. Discussion of the patient's case in the presence of all the persons concerned with his care may be most revealing in that it will bring to light negative as well as positive attitudes of the family.

(3) *Rate of progress of the disorder.* Occasionally a patient is seen at the height of his illness. The fact that he finally agreed to consult a psychiatrist may have been the first sign of incipient recovery, and improvement occurs soon after the first interview. Such encouraging results are only obtained in illnesses of short duration. Much more frequently the patient's condition has been worsening over some time, and the march of events during the weeks or days before consultation is likely to continue afterwards at a similar rate. Therefore, rapid recent increase in the severity of symptoms is a clear danger signal, and points to the need for early admission to hospital.

Determining the rate of progress of a disorder may also help to disentangle the different components of a clinical picture. Where the symptomatology is mainly affective, a fluctuating course may indicate not only phasic variations but also the influence of some external factors, and thus indicate methods of treatment and management. Marked changes from confused to relatively lucid episodes over a number of months, or even years, suggest that a focal or recurrent rather than a global and progressive pathological process is at work, and all that may be required are temporary measures. It is often difficult to decide how much significance to attach to failures in tests of memory and comprehension administered to old people. A history of memory difficulties going back over many years, combined with only slight impairment at the time of the examination, indicates that the progress of mental decline has been very slow, and perhaps in keeping with the patient's age. Depressive or persecutory symptoms may be much more important, and call for energetic treatment. On the other hand, a rapid decline in mental abilities over the past few months makes the presence of definitely pathological brain changes highly probable, especially when associated affective, schizophreniform or neurotic symptoms are mild and variable.

PHYSICAL ASSESSMENT

It is unnecessary to stress the importance of careful and complete physical examinations, and it is not possible to cover in this book the whole subject of geriatric medicine. Severe and obvious physical illnesses are, of course, first seen and treated by general or geriatric physicians and surgeons, who usually attempt to deal with any mental complications, or who will assist with physical diagnosis and treatment when transfer of the patient to psychiatric care becomes necessary. Psychiatrists have to look out for less obvious physical symptoms and signs in patients referred to them directly. There are a number of common and important physical conditions which should be kept in mind when examining an elderly psychiatric patient, because they are known to cause mental symptoms, to affect treatment and to influence the prognosis of psychiatric disorders.

Toxins cause mental symptoms at all ages, but the very young and the very old are most severely affected by them. The fact that excessive alcohol or drugs have been taken by the patient, or that these had been administered to them on doctor's orders, should have been elicited when taking the history. Many of these substances produce fairly characteristic physical signs and mental symptoms. Since the use of bromides and long-acting barbiturates has become obsolete, bacterial and metabolic toxins are far more frequently encountered causes of psychiatric states in the aged. Bacterial toxins usually originate from hidden or inconspicuous foci of infection, the commonest being unsuspected (because afebrile) pneumonic consolidation, and urinary infection. Mildly impaired senile persons may become severely confused as the result of small superficial areas of inflammation, boils, whitlows and even ingrowing toe-nails (examination of the feet is frequently resisted by the elderly!). The commonest metabolic intoxication causing mental symptoms in our age group is uraemia, most often associated with urinary bladder obstruction. Other easily missed metabolic intoxications are those due to mild diabetes, hepatic failure and gout. It is desirable to carry out chest X-rays, urinary analysis and microscopy, as well as examinations of the blood for anaemia, leucocytosis and erythrocyte sedimentation rate in every patient, as these may lead to the discovery of toxic and other conditions which had remained undetected during the physical examination of feeble and uncooperative old persons.

Various deficiencies are also especially prone to occur and to precipitate mental symptoms in old people. Though not officially classed as a deficiency disorder, anoxia may be discussed here. Cerebral anoxia commonly results from cardiac failure and emphysema, acting singly or in combination. Anoxic confusion following severe cardiac infarcts or gastro-intestinal bleeding is usually preceded by a brief period of unconsciousness. The frequency of confusion following surgical anaesthesia has probably been exaggerated. Occlusion or stenosis of the internal carotid arteries were found in some patients who had been looked upon during life as suffering from senile or arteriosclerotic dementia (Fisher, 1951, 1954). Later work showed that only 10–20 per cent of patients with these conditions were dementing, though many more may show milder personality deteriorations (Sours, 1960). Most patients present with cerebral incidents and some type of hemiparesis; many exhibit a Horner's syndrome, but Corsellis and Evans (1963) found that stenosis of neck vessels hardly ever occurred as an isolated phenomenon and apart from vascular cerebral degeneration.

Recent reviews of experimental findings concerning vitamin and hormone deficiencies and treatments have disclosed disappointing results (Inglis, 1958). Frank scurvy, pellagra or beriberi are hardly ever seen in Britain today unless as a secondary result of mental disorder characterised by dietary fads or extreme neglect. Debilitated and neglected old people often improve psychologically as well as physically with vitamin therapy initiated after admission to hospital, but it is then impossible to differentiate any specific effects from those of general nursing, medical and social measures. All the same, it is certainly advisable to be on the look-out for evidence of these deficiencies and for a history of alcoholism. Two deficiency syndromes, which can respond dramatically to treatment, may be difficult to diagnose: psychosis associated with a megaloblastic anaemia or subacute combined degeneration of the spinal cord, and myxoedema.

The occasional unexpected discovery of pernicious anaemia underlines the need for blood examinations in every mentally ill elderly patient. With a complaint of paraesthesiae, and suspected neurological signs, a histamin test-meal and examination of the sternal bone-marrow should be carried out. Many old people look myxoedematous, but it is always worth the trouble, especially when there is a history of voice change, to ask for one of the modern laboratory tests which require minimal co-operation from the patient. Hit-and-miss treatments with iron preparations, vitamin B_{12} injections or thyroid extracts are only excusable in areas without laboratory facilities, as they may delay exact diagnosis for many months.

Physical evidence of brain damage may be obvious, and its relationship to mental illness will occupy us in a later chapter. Thorough and enthusiastic neuropsychiatrists tend to discover neurological abnormalities in most old patients. Mild tremors, rigidities, tics, peripheral absence or diminution of vibration sense, reflex abnormalities limited to one joint, and even a doubtful or positive Babinski response as the only positive neurological finding, should be interpreted in relation to all other clinical features. Doubtful and isolated neurological abnormalities have been shown to lack diagnostic as well as prognostic significance in the overwhelming majority of elderly patients. In view of the atypical symptomatology often found in general paralysis of the insane, in partially treated cases, Wasserman reactions in blood and cerebrospinal fluids have to be tested.

Sensory defects should be carefully assessed in relation to the aetiology and treatment of the psychiatric disorder. The same holds for any other physical disease or disability, as, in the presence of incurable and progressive physical illness, the outlook for a complete and lasting removal of psychiatric symptoms is often poor.

MENTAL STATE

The assessment of the patient's mental state is best carried out on the background of the information obtained from the patient's friends. In the case of in-patients, the observations of the nursing staff are also highly relevant, and, finally, there are the psychiatrist's own impressions and findings on interviewing the patient. As variability from day to day, or even from hour to hour, is an important feature of psychologically disturbed old people, a few days' observation is often desirable in order to arrive at a reliable assessment. At a domiciliary or out-patient consultation, rapid decisions may have to be made concerning immediate management: we have seen that the social impact of the patient's disorder, the rate at which symptoms had recently become more severe, and the presence and nature of any physical illness, were often more important factors determining the action to be taken than a precise psychiatric diagnosis. An experienced clinician may be able to make a correct diagnosis and treatment recommendation in a large proportion of cases at a single consultation. However, doctors less familiar with mental illnesses in old age are advised to take their time. It is a serious mistake to carry out a complete evaluation of a patient in one sitting, and to spend hours with him whilst interviewing him. Various aspects of the patient's condition should be studied as favourable opportunities arise, just as in the examination of a small child. Immediate notes should be taken, but finally a more formal record should be prepared, as is done in general psychiatry, under the following headings: (1) overt behaviour; (2) mood; (3) mental content; and (4) difficulties and disorders of thinking. In the chapters dealing with specific illnesses, abnormalities in any of these areas will be described and discussed fully. Some more general remarks will be made at this stage.

(1) *Overt behaviour* manifests itself in the patient's motor activity, which includes his expressive movements and the form of his talk. In severely disturbed patients, with whom verbal communications are difficult or impossible, skilled observation of all aspects of behaviour may lead to a reasonably good understanding of the nature of the abnormalities present. Impaired awareness betrays itself by a puzzled expression, by wandering around aimlessly, and by repetitive and restless activity. It is likely to be variable, and to be more marked at night, when the patient may attempt to carry out actions appropriate to his home surroundings or to past situations at his work (occupational delirium). The patient's reactions and verbal ejaculations may indicate quite clearly that he is experiencing hallucinations of a visual or auditory type. Restlessness and aggressiveness may sometimes be due to fear and dread, emotions which may also be portrayed in his

facial expression. Less severely disturbed patients may conduct themselves unobtrusively, but inquiry from the nursing staff may elicit that, in fact, they lose their way (especially in relation to their bed and the lavatory), that they misidentify people, that they are unsociable, seclusive and inactive—or the reverse. Information must be obtained about sleep and food intake, and in cases of urinary or faecal incontinence the exact circumstances of these occurrences should be noted.

In many patients abnormalities may only become apparent on interviewing them. Again, facial expression and mobility may tell the observer a good deal; perplexity, anxiety, sadness, emotional empti-ness, or explosive and apparently facile changes from laughing to crying—any of these may yield important leads towards the further exploration of the mental state. The form of the patient's talk, ranging from over-talkativeness and wandering from point to point, to reiterativeness and paucity, and to dysphasic jargon, may be of the greatest diagnostic significance. Clinical examples often lack the typical structure of talk which textbooks give to disorders like flight of ideas, incoherence, anecdotal senile garrulity, or depressive retardation, and a tape recording may prove useful for later analysis.

(2) *Mood disorder* can usually be inferred from the patient's expressive movements, but a full verbal description by the patient allows of a much better evaluation of the presence of euphoria, elation (i.e. feeling of well-being plus increased drive towards activity), sadness, despair, anxiety, tension or loss of feeling. Searching and specific inquiry may be necessary in patients who are initially unable to describe their altered feeling tone, but will only complain of the associated unpleasant somatic sensations (e.g. various abdominal feelings like "butterflies", draggings, thumpings and "turning-over" sensations). Physicians often feel obliged to rule out physical causes for these complaints by laboratory and other investigations, and fail to elicit at an early stage the associated anxiety.

(3) *Exploration of the patient's mental content* should be extensive as well as intensive, taking as a starting base the type of mood and behaviour deviation shown by the patient, as well as the patient's own complaints. His own account of the illness and his ideas concerning causation should be recorded here, and in the case of many paranoid illnesses a complete picture of his thought disorder may emerge. Usually, more searching exploration is required for melancholic and

suicidal thought content, for hypochondriacal, paranoid or grandiose preoccupations, and for obsessive or phobic symptoms. Following this overall assessment, time should be spent (and this may be therapeutic in promoting rapport) on getting as complete a picture as possible of the patient's pathological ideas, experiences and attitudes; e.g. when an affective disorder appears predominant, exploration for hopelessness, guilt, self-reproach, physical symptoms, depersonalization, etc.; or, when a schizophrenic disorder is suspected, for the presence of passivity experiences, bizarre hypochondriasis or intrusions and projections of thought. An attempt should be made to trace out all the ramifications of obsessional or phobic phenomena from the time when they first appeared. Finally, it is important to record the severity of abnormal mental contents and the degree to which the patient is convinced of their reality. Quoting exactly what the patient says is essential here; labels like "delusions", "hallucinations" and "insight" should not be used in clinical records.

It may be objected that in a busy clinic or hospital there is not sufficient time for such complete assessment, and that full notes cannot possibly be made. My answer is that time spent in this way will turn out to be time saved. As we shall see, elderly psychiatric patients need a good deal of treatment and supervision for the rest of their lives, and a full initial record of one's findings will help in interpreting the significance of later occurrences.

(4) *Disorders of thinking processes.* Abnormalities of cognitive functioning may be the result of manic-depressive or schizophrenic disturbances, but most commonly cognitive impairment is due to cerebral dysfunctioning or deterioration. Its assessment will not be informative without knowledge of the subject's past mental abilities—his school history, his work history, the general level of his past achievements. If on this background of information there is a reliable account of failing powers and abilities, or if there is a history of confused wanderings from home, neglect of person or incontinence—in any of these circumstances the presence of severe intellectual impairment can usually be confirmed by a few questions. It may be found that the patient can give her maiden name only, may give an age much younger than her years, claim that her long-deceased parents are still alive, and when asked various dates may perseverate, e.g. on the year of her birth. Every doctor is familiar with this sort of picture.

In many instances, intellectual difficulties are less obvious, and a more searching evaluation is necessary. It is rarely possible to confirm and measure decline in mental abilities in a realistic fashion, e.g. by observing a carpenter in the hospital workshop, or a housewife in the kitchen. As a rule we have to assess patients at the bedside or in our office, with verbal or pencil-and-paper tests. We saw (Chapter I) that the processes of memory and learning tend to be impaired in certain ways with advancing age, but much more seriously in senile mental disorders. Fortunately, memory disorders lend themselves very well to investigation with tests, and for this reason the examination of memory and learning ability has always played an important part in assessing the cognitive functioning of psychiatric patients. My psychological colleagues (Shapiro *et al.*, 1956) examined a number of customary clinical procedures in a group of 100 psychiatric patients over the age of 60. It was found, when proper methodological precautions were taken, that most of the time-honoured so-called sensorium tests failed to differentiate patients with brain damage from those without cerebral pathology. These included the recall of a name and an address, of items of a brief newspaper paragraph, the repetition of a span of digits (forwards and backwards), simple additions and subtractions, and the rendering and comprehension of a brief story. Possibly these tasks were too difficult for mentally disturbed elderly people. By contrast, patients without cerebral pathology scored as a group significantly higher on questionnaires covering dates in their personal lives, and names and events of historical or political significance. Answers to questions concerning orientation for time, place and persons, as well as their ability to learn their way about in the ward, also permitted differentiation (at a statistically acceptable level) of cerebrally disordered from "functional" patients. For some years we have been using the questionnaires which are reprinted with scoring instructions as an appendix to this chapter. The questions covering impersonal events have to be brought up to date from time to time, and could no doubt be adapted for use in other countries. Scores obtained in these questionnaires must not be expected to diagnose individual patients as either "functional" or "organic". In the original study quite a number of organic patients had high, and functional ones low, scores, as differentiation had only been successful in terms of group means. In addition, the ability to answer questions is affected by original intelligence, education, interest and continued ability to take in recent happenings; failure to give correct details of the sovereign, her family, or of recent political events, in the case of a solicitor of 65, who continues to prop up his *The Times* in front of him at breakfast, has far more serious significance than the same degree of failure in a 70-year-old charwoman who has been agitated and depressed during the preceding six months. The main advantage of using these questionnaires lies in the fact that tasks which are too difficult have been excluded, and that a wide area of memory functioning is tapped. Their use may demonstrate that patients remember past events very well, but recent ones very poorly, or that their only failure lies in the area of impersonal memory. Orientation, or learning the spatial layout of the ward may be particularly defective. Though overall performance may be quite good, patchy failure may suggest the presence of focal brain damage or of early generalised cerebral deterioration. Some answers to questions may demonstrate the phenomenon of perseveration: replies to earlier questions being given repeatedly and inappropriately to later ones. Patients may name sovereigns, prime ministers, presidents, and war dates belonging to their younger years, incidentally demonstrating that their inability to give recent dates is not due to a lifelong limited outlook or the result of poor intelligence. Refusal of questions by a series of "don't knows" is commonest in depressed patients. Organically confused or demented people tend to give wrong answers or to produce plausible excuses for their lack of knowledge; they may even be induced to fill the gaps in their memories by imaginary improvisations. This phenomenon (called confabulation) is, like perseveration, very suggestive of organic mental impairment.

Cognitive functions other than memory and learning should be investigated as well, especially when the history suggests the presence of some specific disabilities. It does not take long to ask a patient to name a number of common and less common objects, to get him to read out a passage, to write a few sentences, or to show his grasp of the use of numbers; simple designs may be copied, and a man or a bicycle drawn. A patient may be asked to point to parts and different sides of his body, to carry out some simple tasks, and to indicate how he would do various things. Watching a patient dress and undress is often very instructive. Aphasia, acalculia, finger agnosia, general agnosia, and apraxia, along with memory impairment, can all be demonstrated in a case of advanced and generalised dementia. When any of these disabilities occur in isolation, focal brain disorder may be suspected, and attempts made at localising the trouble by a fuller examination. We are here entering the realm of neurology, and the reader is once again referred to Allison's (1962) book.

In a reasonably co-operative patient it is well within the clinician's competence to obtain estimates of general intelligence, using the Mill Hill Vocabulary Test and Raven's Progressive Matrices (especially the coloured version), which have been standardised for use in elderly people (Raven, 1958a, 1958b). Low scores in these tests in professional people, skilled workers, and persons with past intellectual interests are suggestive of intellectual impairment. Marked discrepancies between scores on the vocabulary rating with those on the performance rating are often found in patients with brain damage.

However, it is important to keep in mind that, taken in isolation, evaluation of a patient's present cognitive status will only tell whether there is some impairment. Certain phenomena like perseveration, telescoping of events, confabulation, and patchiness of performance are suggestive of cerebral disorders, but the significance of defects can only be assessed in relation to all other findings, as impairment may be due to temporary cerebral dysfunctioning, to permanent anatomical brain damage, or to the temporary effects of emotional disturbance. The use of more elaborate psychological tests, of electroencephalography, and of X-ray studies will be described with the proviso that results have to be interpreted in relation to all other findings.

SOME SPECIAL DIAGNOSTIC TECHNIQUES

PSYCHOLOGICAL CONSULTATION

My present view is that projective and interpretative techniques used by clinical psychologists are not sufficiently validated to be employed for routine clinical use; further research may well alter the position. The present discussion will be confined to tests of cognitive impairment, employed by psychologists to measure the same abilities and functions, which are the clinician's concern: various aspects of memory and learning, spatial perception, thought processes, speech function, etc. The psychologist's approach presents a considerable refinement on the clinician's procedures in that the method of administering tests is strictly standardised. Also the results are numerically scored, and have been validated by comparing the performance of a sample of independently diagnosed patients (the criterion group) with that of a suitable matched control group. Unfortunately, there is not a single test of cognitive impairment which will in all circumstances differentiate, without an area of overlapping scores, groups of patients independently diagnosed as brain damaged, from healthy subjects. Therefore, in a given patient the psychologist may not be able to state that he performs like a brain-damaged person, but merely that his score was obtained by a certain proportion of the brain-damaged criterion group, but also by a proportion of members of the control population. We must also remember that even when a patient's score is so low that it falls below the area of overlap, the impairment may not, after all, be due to a pathological process in the brain. After excluding uncooperative subjects, we found that some severely depressed and perplexed elderly people gave scores indicating brain damage on certain learning tests; after successful treatment of the mental illness their scores rose to normal levels (Kendrick *et al.*, 1963).

The clinician who vaguely suspects the presence of a dementing process in a mentally disturbed or slightly failing old man or woman, and who simply orders "tests of deterioration" is bound to be disappointed. In these circumstances the patient's score on various tests is likely to place him in the overlap area between the scores obtained by the original criterion group and the group of normal control subjects, i.e. the psychologist will agree with the clinician in calling the patient "doubtfully impaired"—which is no help. The psychologist may find that the patient's score places him clearly within the criterion group of brain-damaged patients. This confirms the clinician's suspicion, but does not exclude the possibility that the patient's "organic" score is due to depression, anxiety or perplexity. In this situation, a non-ambiguous psychological report that the patient's scores place him within the normal range will probably be the most useful outcome of the investigation, suggesting that the clinician's suspicion has not been confirmed by more reliable methods of cognitive assessment. However, there is a further difficulty; most psychological tests of intellectual deterioration give positive results only in cases of generalised brain damage. Memory and learning ability, as well as general intelligence, may be unimpaired in patients with focal, e.g. parietal lobe lesions; on the other hand, intelligence tests may give normal results in Korsakov's syndrome, when memory and learning functioning may be seriously impaired in isolation. If we add, as a reminder, that doubts as to the presence of a dementing process are often raised in severely disturbed and for this reason untestable patients, we are forced to conclude that psychological testing has a strictly limited scope in the diagnosis of psychiatric disorders of old age. Confirmation of clinically obvious confusion or dementia may occasionally be desirable, though hardly ever necessary; exclusion of the presence of brain damage may sometimes be possible and reassuring; and special tests may help in localising focal disorders, e.g. a marked discrepancy of scores in tests of visual as against auditory learning may confirm the presence of a lesion in a temporal lobe. Psychological tests may turn out to play their most useful role in determining the degree of recovery following a cerebral episode, and in gauging by means of serial testing the rate of progress of dementia in individual patients. We have only just begun to investigate these possibilities. In the present state of our knowledge, clinicians should discuss each diagnostic problem fully with a psychologist in order to discover what help can be given, and psychological tests should never be ordered like serological or biochemical investigations. All the same, it is helpful for the clinician to be conversant with some commonly used tests of generalised brain damage.

After reviewing a considerable number of tests in common use, Yates (1954) concluded: "It is doubtful whether any aspect of psychological testing has been more inadequately treated than the diagnostic assessment of brain damage." The reader will find a more recent discussion of the use of tests in elderly patients in Inglis's (1958) article. Here we shall only discuss procedures which have been found useful in my department in recent years.

(1) *The Bender Visual-Motor Gestalt Test (1938)*. This test consists of nine simple designs, presented successively. The subject is instructed to copy them with a pencil on a piece of paper in front of him. Given in a slightly modified version, this test was found to differentiate elderly patients with "organic" psychoses from elderly "functional" patients at a higher level of statistical significance and with less overlap than any of twenty-four other measures employed, singly or in combination (Shapiro *et al.*, 1956). A scoring method has been devised, and a further study demonstrated that failure to copy designs by organic mental patients was largely due to their relative inaccuracy in copying right angles (Shapiro *et al.*, 1957). The differentiating

power of this test was confirmed in a two-year follow-up of a sample of patients, but the scores failed to predict whether the course of their illness was likely to be relatively benign or malignant (Inglis *et al.*, 1960). With this perceptual-motor test, memory and learning ability play an insignificant part in successful performance. The next test to be mentioned relies on the ability to reproduce information acquired at various times of life.

(2) *The Tooting Bec Questionnaire*. This questionnaire was designed during a study (conducted at the Tooting Bec Hospital, London) correlating oxygen utilisation of elderly dements with their psychometric scores. It was found to correlate just as well as a number of sub-tests of the much more elaborate Wechsler Bellevue Intelligence Scale. The questionnaire (for a full description see Doust *et al.*, 1953) consists of twenty-two items covering information of past and recent personal life events as well as on some political matters. It has not been fully standardised or validated, but was found effective in differentiating with very little overlap, persistently confused subjects between the ages of 70 and 96 from non-confused subjects. Correct answers given on more than nine items excluded the presence of dementia. On the other hand, its presence was confirmed by patients answering correctly only eight or fewer questions (Cosin *et al.*, 1958).

This test, like all other so-called memory questionnaires and scales in use, relies on a person's ability to reproduce information acquired in the past and subsequently stored. It has been shown that performance on memory tests of this type also depends very much on the subject's level of general intelligence. Therefore, Inglis (1957) constructed a learning test which was thought to be as independent as possible of general intellectual functioning, but at the same time sensitive to clinical memory impairment as found in elderly subjects.

(3) *A Paired-Associate Learning Test for use in elderly psychiatric patients* (*Inglis, 1957*). The PALT may be presented auditorily or visually in a number of equivalent forms. In each there are three stimulus words and, associated with them, three response words to be learnt by the patient; e.g. in Form A:

	Stimulus	*Response*
(*a*)	Cabbage	Pen
(*b*)	Knife	Chimney
(*c*)	Sponge	Trumpet

After an initial explanation, including a trial run with similar material, the patient is asked, following the first presentation, to give the correct response word after the examiner has offered the stimulus word: "What went with 'knife'?" The presentation of the stimulus words in random order is continued until each of the three responses is given correctly three times running. The test is abandoned if this criterion is not reached after each stimulus word has been presented thirty times. The score is simply the total number of repetitions required until learning has occurred: i.e. ranging from 3 points for learning at the first presentation, to 93 points for failure to learn after 3 times 30 further trials.

In the original experiment, eighteen patients with severe and definite memory impairment were matched for age and intelligence scores with eighteen patients without clinically discernible memory difficulties, and none of the latter required more than twenty-eight trials before learning, to the criterion of three consecutive correct repetitions of all three response words. Only one of the memory-impaired patients had a lower score. Parsons (1962), during a survey of a random sample of old people living in their own homes, found the following:

Psychiatric assessment	N	Mean PALT score
Normal memory	141	17·4
Slightly impaired	48	23·1
Definitely forgetful	19	42·3
Severely demented	6	81·2

It is suggested that this learning test measures impairment of the acquisition phase of memory function, which involves short-term storage of information. This is a mechanism whose importance in mental ageing was discussed in Chapter I. As the overwhelming majority of cerebral-organic disorders in old age are associated with deterioration of memory, the presence of a dementing process will, in practice, be indicated by a score on the PALT which is higher than thirty trials. Experience suggests, however, that for subjects tested outside a hospital setting it may be wiser to accept as within normal limits a score below 40. As with other tests of cognitive impairment, abnormally high scores may also be obtained in temporarily confused or severely perplexed and depressed patients.

(4) *The Modified Word Learning Test* (*Walton and Black, 1957, 1958*). This test is based on the finding that persons with generalised brain damage tend to have undue difficulties in learning the meaning of words with which they are unfamiliar (Shapiro and Nelson, 1955). In administering the test, the patient is first given the vocabulary section of an intelligence test and then asked to learn the meanings of the first ten words which he had been unable to define. These ten new words are gone over with him until the patient is able to give correctly the meaning of six. His score is obtained by subtracting from 11 the number of times the definitions had to be repeated. Thus, a patient who learns the meaning of six words on the first presentation scores 10 points; when one repetition is required, the score is 9 points, and so on.

In the validation study, no normal, neurotic or functionally psychotic subject obtained a score lower than 6, and 97·1 per cent of brain-damaged patients were correctly identified by a score of 5 or under. This test may not pick out patients with focal brain damage, and persons of low intelligence may give false "organic" scores. Certain modifications have been suggested for use in geriatric patients (Kendrick *et al.*, 1963).

Other useful psychological tests of cognitive impairment include the Graham–Kendall Memory for Design Test (1960, 1962) and the Minnesota Percepto-Diagnostic Test (1963).

ELECTROENCEPHALOGRAPHY

Monitoring cerebral activity by electrical means might be thought of considerable value in tracing some psychological disturbances back to cerebral dysfunctioning. Unfortunately, experience has shown that, for the present, electroencephalography has only limited applications in the clinical psychiatry of old age. There are several reasons for this. Only a small proportion of cerebral tissue, lying immediately underneath a thick covering of skull and scalp, is accessible to electrical exploration. Abnormal discharges derive only from damaged or dying tissues, and atrophied areas of the brain are probably electrically silent. Electrical sampling of accessible areas can only be carried out over relatively short periods. Finally, wide divergencies of opinion still exist among experts as to the significance of various phenomena, and there is also a good deal of uncertainty regarding normal and abnormal age changes in the electroencephalogram.

Frey and Sjoegren (1959) have summarised the position as follows: *Alpha rhythm:* during the first twenty years of life the average alpha frequency is said to rise rapidly to about 9 cycles/second, but then more slowly to 10·5 c/s. After or just before the age of 60, this frequency again begins to drop slightly. Possibly a frequency of 8·5 c/s at 70 corresponds to one of 9·5 c/s in a person of 30. Slowing or disappearance of alpha rhythms is more commonly seen in demented as against non-organic psychotic elderly people. *Theta-activity* (4–7 c/s) is present more often in psychotics who have epileptic seizures, and in demented patients. *Beta-activity* (14–25 c/s): opinions are said to vary. Some say that this is more frequently found with increasing age, but others deny this. In quoted authors' opinion, it appeared to be significantly diminished in patients with dementia, with the suggestion that the absence of beta-activity might be due to cortical atrophy. *Delta-activity* (0·5–3·5 c/s): bursts of low frequency activity occurred mainly in demented subjects. *Focal activities* have been described in 20–30 per cent of elderly control subjects. They are most frequently seen in patients with neurological signs (see also Silverman *et al.*, 1955). There is a suggestion that severely demented seniles with a short expectation of life have significantly more severe EEG abnormalities (especially low frequency activities) than less seriously demented patients with longer average periods of survival.

Turning to the question of differential diagnosis, it has been found that there is good correlation between a clinical diagnosis of severe and definite dementia and the presence of severe EEG changes. However, cases of this type do not normally pose a clinical problem. On the other hand, there tends to be only poor correlation between EEG slow wave changes that are not gross, and a clinical diagnosis of dementia which is not severe. "Hence, the EEG is not a satisfactory weapon for routine use in attempting to assess the degree of early dementia in 'mixed' cases, where affective components are also present, and ordinary psychiatric judgment still appears the soundest diagnostic and prognostic approach" (Turton, 1958). We came to the same conclusion in a study comparing clinical diagnosis, independent EEG findings and outcome assessed two years later. In patients where the clinician had been doubtful about the presence of a cerebral disorder, EEG findings failed to give correct prognostic indications, except very occasionally (Pampiglione and Post, 1958).

The present position of electroencephalography in the psychiatry of old age was recently reviewed in a summary article by Hill and Driver (1962). They state categorically that EEG patterns do not relate to irreversible deterioration in cognitive ability. They go on to say that most demented patients (pre-senile, senile and arteriosclerotic) whose dementia is not associated with epileptiform fits or dependent on either a tumour or a rapidly developing cerebral disease with oedema, have normal EEGs. They also deny that there is any relationship between the EEG and the clinical picture in Alzheimer's pre-senile dementia. Here, as in other forms of dementia, the EEG picture is related to the rapidity of progress of the illness rather than to specific histological changes.

In summary, electroencephalographic examinations of elderly patients cannot be expected to prove useful in solving difficult diagnostic problems, but the amount and type of abnormal electrical activity, taken together with other clinical features, may indicate the rate and severity of any pathological cerebral process present. A constant slow wave focal abnormality, particularly with irregular wave form, should always suggest the presence of a space-occupying expanding lesion which demands further neurological investigation.

PNEUMOENCEPHALOGRAPHY

It is usually said that in senile and pre-senile dementias the sulci of the brain are widened and the ventricles dilated. There are, however, no reliable recent studies which compare the brains of dements with those of mentally normal old people, though there is a strong impression that some degree of cerebral atrophy becomes increasingly common with rising age (see also Chapter III). There are also no publications comparing the configuration of the brain and its ventricles visualised by X-ray studies during life with the appearances at post-mortem.

Writers of textbooks give the warning that radiologically apparent cerebral atrophy is not necessarily indicative of a dementing illness. In fact Gosling (1955) found that atrophy was shown in the air-pictures of 11 per cent of 213 non-demented persons over 45; on the other hand, 15 per cent of 68 senile and pre-senile dements had normal lumbar pneumoencephalograms. In his study he did not rely only on visual impressions, but also on various measurements of the X-ray film.

McCormick (1962) found that for technical reasons (e.g. difficulties in positioning the heads of old people with restricted neck movements) only three kinds of measurements could be obtained from their air-pictures in almost all the 37 cases of his series of psychiatric patients over the age of 60; (1) the transverse diameter of the anterior horns of the lateral ventricles, which was called normal if it did not exceed 2·1 cm (Plate I); (2) the width of the sulci (normal if not exceeding 0·3 cm (Plate II); (3) the diameter of the third ventricle (normal if not wider than 0·8 cm (Plate III). On the basis of a comprehensive clinical assessment, which included the use of some simple behaviour ratings and psychological tests, patients were graded as not demented, mildly demented, moderately demented and severely demented.

In this sample there was no significant increase of radiologically diagnosed cerebral atrophy with increasing age. A significant correlation between radiological atrophy and degree of dementia was found to exist in only a few comparisons between ratings of dementia and measurements obtained from the AEGs. Most disappointingly, it was not possible to differentiate between patients without dementia and with mild dementia on the basis of the anterior horn diameter, or of this measurement in combination with that of the sulci and of the third ventricle. A value was determined for the sum of these three measurements which permitted 24 of 31 cases to be placed correctly in one of two groups: mildly or not demented, as against moderately or severely demented. The same differentiation could be made correctly in 27 of 37 cases by selecting as a cut-off point, an anterior horn diameter of 3·0 cm. Five of eighteen patients without or with only mild dementia had anterior horn diameters of 3·1 cm or more, whereas 5 of 19 cases had been found definitely demented even though their anterior horns measured only 3·0 cm or less. On account of this degree of misclassification, McCormick concluded that lumbar pneumoencephalography could not be used as a diagnostic tool for the diagnosis of dementia in individual patients.

As this is an unpleasant experience for the patient, which also carries a small but definite mortality risk, air-encephalography should only be employed when the presence of a space-occupying lesion is suspected. I feel it is also indicated in relatively young geriatric patients, under the age of 70 or thereabouts, with recently developed dementia without obvious cerebrovascular causation. Beyond this age, the chances of discovering an operable tumour as against merely confirming global dementia become infinitesimally small.

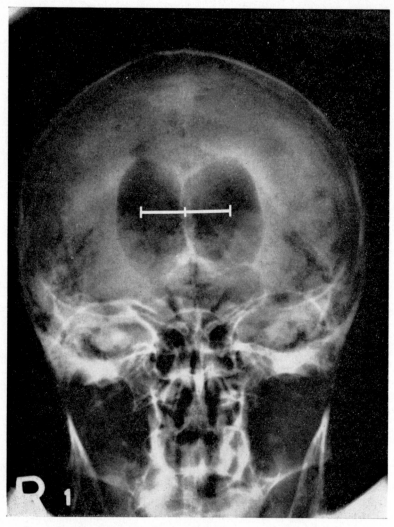

PLATE I. Dilated anterior horns of lateral ventricles. (Normal width of
2·1 cm as indicated.)

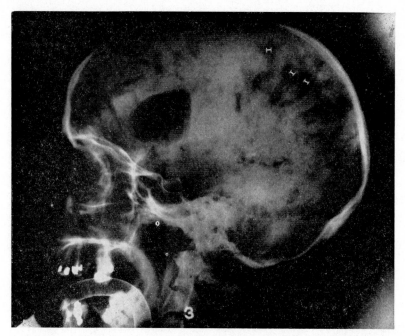

PLATE II. Dilated cerebral sulci. (Normal width of 0·3 cm as indicated.)

FINAL REMARKS

In the following chapters, different kinds of psychiatric disorders commonly seen in elderly people will have to be described and discussed separately in spite of our earlier expressed view that psychiatric diagnostic classifications are at the present time only provisional at all ages. Moreover, in the elderly both physical and psychological disorders are usually present at the same time, one influencing the other. Psychiatric symptomatology tends to present as a composite picture, made up of the following: the effects of "normal" and "abnormal" ageing especially of the nervous and endocrine systems, inherited and acquired personality structure, constitutional mental reaction type (e.g. schizophrenic or affective), and past and present social factors in the widest sense of the word.

At the beginning of an illness, precise diagnosis and correct prognosis are, therefore, rarely feasible. It is more important and

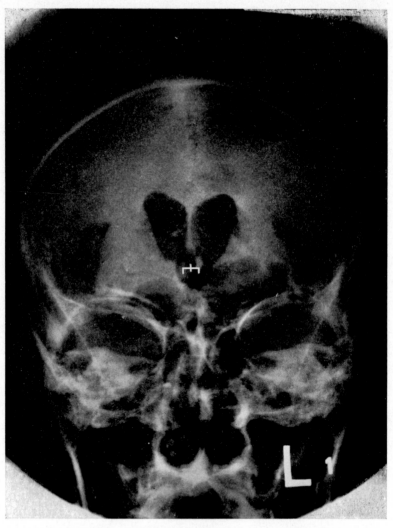

PLATE III. Dilated third ventricle. (Normal diameter of 0·8 cm as indicated.)

realistic to discover the past duration of a disorder and its rate of progress. Where the disorder is well established, findings obtained on physical and mental examination, as well as by special tests and investigations will confirm diagnostic formulations. In patients with more recent illnesses, each finding has to be interpreted in the light of all the other clinical data, especially the history of the patient's life and illness.

GENERAL ORIENTATION[1]

Initials of Dr.............................. Date.............................. Time..............................

Score   Question   Verbatim answer

Where are you now?

What is this place called?

Where is it situated?

What day of the week is it today?

What month are we in?

What day of the month is it?

What is the year?

What time is it? (allow 30 min deviation to score.)

Score leniently 1 point for each question answered correctly.

Total score   Maximum score 8.

---

[1] These questionnaires, except the last one, should be administered some 3–4 days following admission.

MEMORY FOR PAST PERSONAL EVENTS

Initials of Dr................................ Date................................ Time................................

Score   Question   Verbatim answer

Where were you born?

What year were you born? (Exact year to score.)

How old were you when you left school?

What year did you get married? (If unmarried, what year did you leave home?) (Actual year has to be given to score.)

Where was your first employment? (Rough indication such as "a family in Clapham", "a factory in Leeds", etc., accepted.)

How many years since you were last employed? (If still employed, how many years have you been in this job?) ("Not since the war" or "Not since I got married", etc., accepted.)

When were you last in hospital? (1 point either for exact year *or* "three years ago" or something like that.)

When did your mother die?

How many jobs have you had? (Rough estimate may do, but not too marked deviation—such as 10 jobs if 15 in actual fact.)

When was your first child born? (If unmarried, birthday of one of your brothers or sisters.) Actual year has to be given for scoring.

What is the name of the school you went to?

How old were you when you got married? (If unmarried, how old were you when you left home?) Exact age for scoring.

Total score   Deviation within a few years, i.e. 1–2 years allowed for scoring.

Re 5 and 6: if patient never had any employment, do not score *both* 5 and 6.

Maximum score 12.

MEMORY FOR RECENT PERSONAL EVENTS

Initials of Dr............................... Date............................... Time...............................

Score	Question	Verbatim answer

When were you admitted to this hospital? (Date and day of week.)

How did you get here? (Form of transport and route.) 1 point if either correct. 2 points if both correct.

Did anybody accompany you? Who? 1 point for correct answer.

Did you see another doctor before you came here? (Not G.P.) Name? 1 point only—only if name given.

Where did you see him and when? 1 point if either indicated. 2 points if both; exact name of place has to be given for scoring. *Re* time, such statement as "last month", etc., will do for scoring.

What is my name? (Make sure you introduce yourself to patient once or twice during previous interviews.) 1 point only if exact.

When did I last see you? 1 point only if correct.

How many days ago did I take a blood test? (Or, did I take your blood pressure?) 1 point only if correct day is given.

Total score　　　Maximum score 11.

MEMORY FOR GENERAL EVENTS

Initials of Dr........................... Date........................... Time...........................

Score	Question	Verbatim answer

Has anything important happened in the world recently? (Score 1 point for important event, making allowances for patient's educational background.)

Who is on the throne? How many children has she got? What are their names? (1 point for number, and another point if all 4 names correct.)

What is the name of the present Prime Minister?

Who was the Prime Minister before him?

What is the name of the President of the U.S.A.?

Who was the President before him?

When was the last war started/finished? (2 points for both years; 1 point for one year correct.)

Nature of a recent strike, and when was it? (If no response, ask for last big accident or natural catastrophe.) (2 points if *both* reasonably correct.)

Total score   Maximum score 12.

WARD ORIENTATION

To be administered not earlier than one week after patient has been up and about; take patient round the ward.

Initials of Dr.. Date.. Time..

Score	Question	Brief description of abnormal responses
	Where do you sleep?	
	Show me the nearest lavatory.	
	Where do you hang your coat?	
	Where is the dining-room?	
	Where is the bathroom?	
	Where is the main entrance?	
	Are there any other ways out? Where?	
	Show me the dormitories.	
	Where is the television?	
	Where is the nurse's office?	
	What is the name of the nurse in charge of the ward?	
	Who sleeps in the same room with you? (Or next door.)	
	Tell me the names of all the other patients you know. (Score 1 point for each correct name.)	
	Do you know the name of any other doctors or nurses? (Score 1 point for each correct name.)	

Total score

CHAPTER III

DISORDERS ASSOCIATED WITH BRAIN CHANGES

INTRODUCTION

At all ages there are essentially two different types of organic mental reaction: (1) transitory changes in awareness and disorders of experiencing and behaving (acute or sub-acute confusional states, acute brain syndromes), and (2) permanent and irreversible decline of all mental abilities (dementia, chronic brain syndrome). Both syndromes may be the result of traumatic, toxic, metabolic, inflammatory, neoplastic or degenerative brain changes. Any of them may affect elderly people, and in the preceding chapter certain clinical features were pointed out which suggest the presence of disorders such as sub-acute combined degeneration, space occupying lesions, syphilitic infections, etc. Here, we will only deal with those organic mental disorders which characteristically occur late in life: the acute senile confusional states and the dementias of old age. The physical pathology of these disorders will be briefly summarised first.

MORBID ANATOMY

(1) *Acute senile confusional states* (a variety of the acute brain syndrome) may terminate with complete mental recovery, may lead to death from the causative or complicating physical illness, or may herald a dementing process. Post-mortem findings will, therefore, reflect the effects of more than one disorder, and I have not been able to find any clear statement in the literature on the pathology of these essentially transitory conditions. Obviously the most important phenomena are biochemical ones: transitory anoxias of various

types, the effects of bacterial toxins and of abnormal accumulations of metabolites, especially those of glucose.

In acute senile delirium there are, however, no constant or well-defined pathological findings, and the changes that have at times been described are similar in kind to the reactions found in younger subjects suffering from severe general disease, fatigue or vitamin deficiencies; they are reversible under favourable conditions.

(2) *Arteriosclerotic dementia* will result after there has occurred a number of cerebrovascular accidents producing multiple areas of

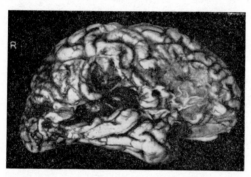

PLATE IV. Right-sided infarction of middle cerebral artery resulting in arteriosclerotic cerebral softening.

cerebral softening (Plate IV). But quite often there are only micro-scopic lesions indicating poor nutrition of the grey matter due to narrowing of smaller vessels (Plate V). Especially in hypertension, temporary insufficiency of cerebral blood supply may be precipitated by general diseases, alcoholism and perhaps also by emotional upsets. So here we have the pathology of one type of acute confusional state. Similarly, after strokes the initial oedema around the area of infarction may subside, and confusional symptoms may disappear with full recovery of mental abilities, at least for the time being. We noted earlier (Chapter II) that interference with cerebral blood supply may also be caused by an obstructive lesion of the internal carotid arteries. Many brains show arteriosclerotic areas of infarction or cell degeneration and glial proliferation, and at the same time parenchymal changes of a senile type. For this reason a clear-cut pathological differentiation between arteriosclerotic and senile dementia is not possible in a proportion of cases.

(3) *Senile Parkinsonism* is seen either as a result of generalized cerebral arteriosclerosis or in paralysis agitans, when degenerative lesions are confined to the substantia nigra, locus caeruleus, globus pallidus and striate body. The main histological findings are atrophy and degeneration of nerve cells, many of which contain inclusion

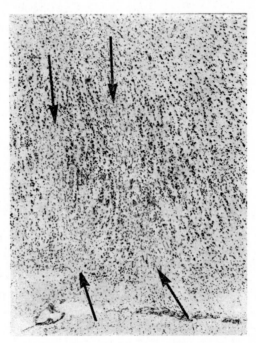

PLATE V. Cerebral cortex showing streaky areas of nerve-cell loss (between arrows) due to impaired blood supply in the diffuse form of cerebral arteriosclerosis.

bodies mainly of hyaline type. The relationship of Parkinsonism to depression and emotional lability is far from clear.

(4) *Senile dementia and Alzheimer's disease*. The pathological appearances in these two conditions are so similar that many workers believe them to be one and the same disease. This controversial issue is fully discussed by McMenemey (1958), and we shall point out later on that there are certain clinical differences between cases of pre-senile dementia (Alzheimer type) starting before the ages of 60–65, and of senile dementia commencing at a later age. Moreover, Larson

et al. (1963) found that no cases of Alzheimer's disease occurred in the families of senile dements, suggesting that these disorders differed genetically. The pathological changes are more severe in cases with early onset, possibly because younger patients tend to live longer in spite of cerebral deterioration, or because in them all pathological processes are more vigorous.

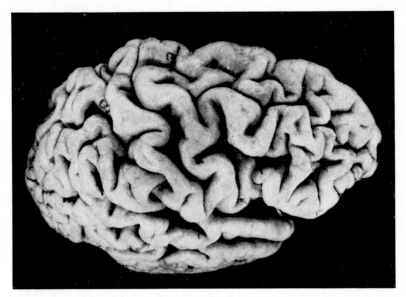

PLATE VI. Cerebral atrophy in senile dementia.

Macroscopically the brain shows generalised atrophy, usually most obviously in the frontal and occipital areas (Plates VI, VII and VIII). On section, the ventricles are generally dilated and the cerebral cortex reduced in thickness. In patients dying early in the disease, macroscopic changes may be inconspicuous. In severe cases, all three of the following histological features will be prominent: (1) severe loss of neurones, especially in layers 3 and 5 of the cerebral cortex; (2) neurofibrillary degeneration of nerve cells; and (3) striking numbers of argyrophilic plaques (Plate IX). The significance of these two structures, their composition, origin and relationship to normal and pathological ageing—all these are still matters of considerable doubt and conjecture (see McMenemey, 1958).

3

(5) *Pick's disease* is a type of pre-senile dementia (but may occur after the age of 65) which usually commences earlier than Alzheimer's disease. When it is at all advanced, marked localised cerebral atrophy is obvious. This is generally confined to the frontal and temporal lobes, and may be asymmetrical. Moreover, the onto-genetically older parts of these lobes, e.g. the posterior two-thirds of the superior temporal gyrus, tend to be spared. Atrophy is not

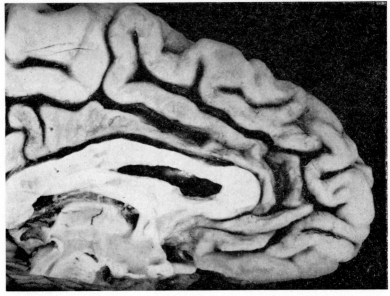

PLATE VII. Atrophy of medial surface of frontal lobe.

confined to the cortex, and shrinkage of the white matter of the affected lobes is a constant feature.

Histological changes are strictly confined to the atrophied portions of the brain. There is loss of nerve cells, and cortical as well as subcortical gliosis, perhaps secondary to the disappearance of neurones. The presence of Pick cells is characteristic of the disorder. They show a peculiar type of cell-swelling with an accumulation of weakly acidophylic protein material displacing the nucleus, and sometimes flattening it, against the cell membrane (Plate X). Senile plaques and neurofibrillary changes may also be found, but again only in the atrophied portions of the brain.

Brief mention should be made of some even rarer pre-senile dementias grouped under the name of *Creutzfeld–Jacob disease*. These conditions are characterised by rapidly progressive dementia in association with Parkinsonism and amyotrophy. Usually there has been insufficient time for cerebral atrophy to occur, but there is severe nerve-cell loss throughout the brain and the cord; other nerve cells may be swollen with lipochrome.

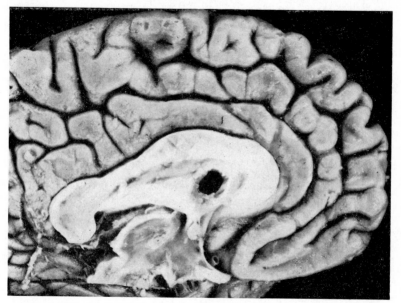

PLATE VIII. Medial surface of normal frontal lobe (for comparison with Plate VI).

(6) *The pathological anatomy of memory.* Memory dysfunction, especially of learning and of reproducing unfamiliar material, is the leading early symptom of most dementing illnesses of late life. By taking account of the localised lesions in Wernicke's encephalopathy, which frequently forms the pathological basis of Korsakoff's syndrome, of observations in temporal lobe surgery, and of findings in cases of subacute encephalitis, Brierley (1961) demonstrated "that a relatively small group of structures are essential to the process of memorising. They fall into two zones, a posterior or cortical comprising the hippocampi . . . and the hippocampal gyri . . . and an

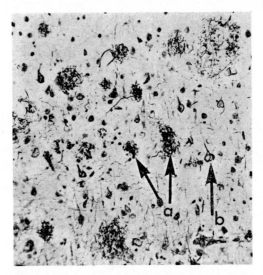

PLATE IX. Silver impregnation of cerebral cortex showing senile plaques
(a) and Alzheimer's neurofibrillary change (b).

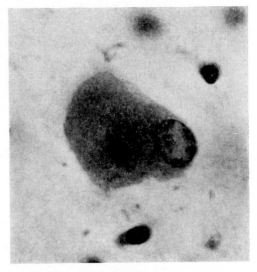

PLATE X. Swollen nerve cell often seen in Pick's disease.

anterior or hypothalamic consisting of the mammillary bodies of the posterior hypothalamus." The fornix is the main pathway connecting these two zones with one another, but their connections with the rest of the brain have not as yet been clearly established. It has been suggested by Penfield's electrical stimulation experiment that the outer and under aspects of the temporal lobes constitute a storehouse of past memories. However, the present position is that memory has no localisation, but that intact hippocampal and mammillary zones are essential for the process of memorising.

Brierley goes on to point out that in many reported instances of arteriosclerotic and senile (Alzheimer's) dementia with marked memory disorder, arteriosclerotic lesions, senile plaques and neuro-fibrillary changes have been found to affect especially severely the ammon's horns, hippocampal gyri and mammillary bodies. By contrast, in Pick's disease, it is usual for the ontogenetically older parts of the temporal lobes containing the hippocampi and the hippocampal gyri to be spared. Relative preservation of certain aspects of memory function, in spite of severe dysphasia, has often been demonstrated in patients with this disorder.

SYMPTOMATOLOGY

GENERAL MATTERS

In describing and discussing various clinical pictures, I propose to adopt the modern approach to the psychiatry of brain disease as summarised by Manfred Bleuler (1954). It is briefly this: with a few exceptions (certain types of poisoning) mental symptoms are no longer regarded as specific to the localisation and cause of brain damage, but the psychic disturbances are thought to be related in a much more general fashion to the extent of pathological brain changes and to the rate with which they develop. We shall see, later on in this chapter, that previous personality and mental health help to shape the clinical picture in a pathoplastic fashion, but first of all we shall demonstrate, with the aid of a diagram (Plate XI), the relationship between the most commonly seen pathogenic events in the brain and the different types of organic mental disorder.

(A) Here we have a suddenly or fairly rapidly occurring lesion, most often due to a minor cerebrovascular accident, which may result in a permanent neurological defect, but which need not have any direct psychological consequences.

(B) An equally sudden but larger lesion is likely to be followed by a period of unconsciousness. On coming to, the patient may pass through an acute confusional state (e.g. post-traumatic delirium following cerebral contusion). This may be followed by complete restoration of mental normality, but there are likely to be some

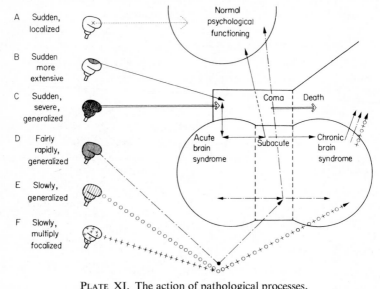

PLATE XI. The action of pathological processes.

neurological defects. By far the commonest event of this kind, in the elderly, is, of course, a stroke. When there has resulted a large area of infarction, and especially when the event is repeated, mental sequelae of a permanent sort—dementia (chronic brain syndrome) will result. The possibility that death may occur at any stage in this and the other examples has not been repeatedly indicated in the diagram in order to preserve clarity.

(C) When the cerebral insult is very severe, generalised and sudden, deep coma is likely to be followed by death (e.g. in the case of severe infarctions or cerebral haemorrhages).

(D) Here the brain is affected globally and fairly rapidly by either of two kinds of processes: (1) mechanical—increase of intracranial pressure due to new growth or subdural haematoma, or (2) bio-chemical—anoxia, deficiencies or diffusion of toxic substances. With both sources of disturbance there is likely to result an acute or sub-acute confusional state, often with marked fluctuations. Outcome clearly depends on the extent to which the pathological events are reversible—complete recovery, residual mental impairment amounting to a permanent defect, or death.

(E) Generalised brain damage occurs slowly and diffusely over wide areas of the brain, most commonly in senile or pre-senile dementia, and a chronic brain syndrome becomes established without any preliminary acute episodes.

(F) Dementia is produced by slowly developing multiple foci of cerebral degeneration, mainly in the diffuse type of cerebral arteriosclerosis damaging small vessels.

In clinical practice, patients often show a mixture of these happenings, and acute events (A) to (D) are apt to complicate the slowly progressive conditions (E) and (F), with acute confusional states being superadded on dementia.

Acute senile confusional state (*senile delirium*) is the name often given to the acute mental reaction type (acute brain syndrome) as seen in old age. Every doctor is familiar with this condition, and there is no need to quote case records. The disturbance is due to widespread and rapidly developing interference with cerebral functioning, due as we saw (D) to mechanical causes like tumours or haematoma, to toxic substances or abnormal metabolites, or associated with anoxia and other deficiencies. Large cerebral infarcts and the oedema surrounding them are other causes (B). In these cases there may be a sudden disruption of cerebral functioning resulting in unconsciousness, but when the onset is more gradual, extending over a few hours or a day or two, a state of diminished awareness becomes established, with marked variations in its intensity. At times the patient may sink into a subcomatose condition from which he is difficult to rouse; at others his level of consciousness may appear almost normal. This is more likely to occur in subacute confusional states. There may be periods when the patient can be reached and will respond to commands and questions. However, his answers are likely to reveal that he is disorientated, believing himself to be in different surroundings and mistaking the identity of people around him. Behaviour disorders exceeding mild restlessness may bring the patient into psychiatric care. During quiet periods he may exhibit a dazed expression and gaze vacantly about him, but sooner or later there will be outbursts of shouting, often stereotyped repetitions of one or two words, and of severe restlessness and aggressiveness in response to attempts at restraint. The patient is probably severely frightened, but it is not usually possible to tell whether this is due to disorientation and misinterpretations, or whether it is a response to fearful visual hallucinations.

Death from exhaustion or from the underlying physical illness is reported to occur in about 40 per cent of these patients. In the remainder, complete mental recovery is said to be the rule, but hardly any long-term follow-up studies are available in spite of the alleged frequency of the condition. Avery (1945) followed twenty-two patients who made good recoveries from acute senile confusional states, which were the first manifestations of mental changes. Only four were known to be alive without showing any serious senile changes, and eight later suffered from a typical dementia and died. Roth (1955) and his co-workers found that only 26 of 318 consecutive mental hospital patients over 60 suffered from acute confusional states. High immediate death rate and, alternatively, high discharge rate, differentiated them strikingly from senile and arteriosclerotic dements; but the mental states of the twelve patients who were still alive and out of hospital two years later are not given.

Many senile acute and subacute confusional states differ little in causation, course and treatment from those seen at younger ages, i.e. when they are due to cerebral neoplasms and infarcts, cardiac insufficiency, uraemia, severe anaemia, alcoholism or subacute combined degeneration. No doubt some of these conditions are most frequently seen in elderly persons. It should be especially remembered that they are prone to develop subdural haematomas after quite trivial head trauma. Anaesthetics, operations, blindfolding in ophthalmic procedures, bereavements and removal from home are other causes operating especially in the senium. When temporary confusion occurs in relation to cryptic or slight physical disturbances, or when no cause can be found on fullest investigation, I am, contrary to current clinical teaching, inclined to assume the presence of a slowly progressive and as yet mild senile deteriorative process. Possibly some future investigations, more searching than those quoted above, may prove me wrong, but here is a typical case record:

Mrs. K., a part-time cleaner, *aet.* 72, was admitted via a mental observation ward. Her earlier history proved irrelevant, and no abnormality was noted by her family until 4 days before she was brought in for observation. She had become restless during the day and sleepless at night. On several occasions she got up at 1 or 2 a.m., and with an imaginary broom and mop had been found busying herself all over the house ("occupational delirium"). Once or twice she had attempted to get dressed, thinking it was time to get up. Especially at night, she had been pointing to the mantelpiece asking what the little coloured men and women were doing there ("Lilliputian hallucinations"). In the observation ward none of these phenomena were observed, but she was confused and disorientated. No abnormal physical signs were detected and her temperature was normal. After transfer she was at first bewildered, but only occasionally uncertain of her surroundings and of the identity of persons. A few days later no mental abnormality was any longer discoverable. Her performance on cognitive and memory tasks was poor, but seemed not out of keeping with her background. A chest X-ray revealed a small area of resolving pulmonary consolidation, which later on cleared completely. Accordingly, a diagnosis of subacute confusional state secondary to afebrile pneumonia was made. However, two years later she was brought to the out-patient clinic. She had never returned to work, and had been increasingly unable to do her own housework. She had deteriorated in memory and habits, and was found so severely demented that, in view of her social circumstances, institutional care had to be recommended.

More frequently, acute confusional states occur in a setting of well-advanced dementia; they are usually precipitated by some intercurrent physical disease and tend to turn out a terminal event.

THE DEMENTIAS OF OLD AGE

Even at post-mortem, differentiation between the various types of these disorders may be impossible. Sometimes a brain will show purely senile changes, at others there may only be evidence of old or recent cerebrovascular accidents or of diffuse, microscopically focalised arteriosclerotic changes. Quite often, in perhaps 20 per cent of cases (Corsellis, 1962), senile and arteriosclerotic processes appear to have been at work simultaneously. Most pathologists are doubtful whether any valid histological distinction can be made between senile dementia and Alzheimer's pre-senile dementia. Clinicians have shown repeatedly that there are no reliable criteria, clinically differentiating Alzheimer's from Pick's disease in spite of clear-cut anatomical differences. All the same, there are a number of practical considerations making clinical differentiation between various types of dementia desirable.

The recognition of dementia on the basis of history and mental state has been fully dealt with in Chapter II, and we shall assume that in a given case the presence of an irreversible, dementing process has been confirmed as the main source of the mental disorder. When the patient is over the age of 70–75, and especially where there is a long history of mental decline, the cause of dementia is most likely a senile or cerebroarteriosclerotic process, and the presence of a disorder which can be arrested is most unlikely. With a history of strokes, as well as of hypertension or variable blood pressure, vascular disease is likely to have played an important part, and where there is a history of recovery from previous episodes of more severe mental disturbance, one may hope for yet another partial remission. The presence of multiple focal brain damage may be indicated by a mixture of neurological abnormalities: monoplegias, hemiplegias, pseudobulbar paresis, dysphasic symptoms, etc. In the absence of any of these phenomena, senile dementia characterised by a relentlessly progressive course is much more likely to be present, especially when the patient is over 80.

By contrast, in patients below the age of 70–75 with incipient or even with well-established dementia, full medical investigation is usually called for, especially when the condition has developed fairly rapidly, say in the course of one or two years, and when the patient is only in his early sixties. Cerebrovascular disease, senile dementia, or pre-senile dementia (arbitrarily characterised by an onset before the age of 60) are still by far the commonest conditions encountered; however, unless multiple and scattered neurological lesions, a high blood pressure, or renal disease point unequivocally to the presence of cerebrovascular pathology, other possibilities should be excluded. The appearance of the patient may suggest myxoedema or anaemia, which will have to be investigated. Even in the absence of convincing neurological signs, subacute combined degeneration may cause dementia through subcortical lesions. Epileptiform convulsions and various types of dysphasia, dyspraxia and agnosia occur, not only in cerebral arteriosclerosis but also in Alzheimer's disease, cerebral tumours and cerebral neurosyphilis, including GPI, to mention only the commonest possibilities. At an early stage these disorders are not necessarily associated with any physical signs.

In pre-senile dementias, schizophreniform or depressive symptoms sometimes mask intellectual decline. Parietal lobe symptoms, like finger agnosia and acalculia, as well as other types of agnosia, apraxia and dysphasia, are suggestive of the Alzheimer type. Claims that patients with Pick's disease tend to repeat words or brief phrases in a stereotyped fashion, and that they are less restless and hyperkinetic than those with Alzheimer's pre-senile dementia, have not been generally confirmed. Senile dementia tends to develop more slowly, with loss of memory and interests as the leading symptoms, while persecutory or depressive aspects tend to be absent or later symptoms.

Regardless of type, the final clinical pictures of advanced dementia merge indistinguishably one into the other. Patients become unable to carry out the simplest, familiar tasks such as dressing and feeding themselves. Speech dilapidates after passing through a phase of incoherence. Emotional incontinence, labile laughing and crying, explosive rages, etc., give way to an empty facial expression no longer communicating any affective changes. Grasp and sucking reflexes can frequently be elicited. Incontinence of urine and faeces occur sooner or later even in well-nursed and well-supervised patients who become bedridden, increasingly debilitated, and who die from a variety of intercurrent diseases. Toxic or other somatic factors may precipitate a more turbulent terminal acute confusional state. The duration of dementias of old age varies from many years to a few months, and it is not possible to give valid estimates of likely further length of life. A poor physical state, faecal incontinence and total inability in dressing and feeding all indicate early death.

PSYCHOPATHOLOGY

Studies of psychological mechanisms operating in elderly patients with organic psychoses have been carried out by a number of workers in an attempt to gain a closer understanding of the behaviour of patients with these disorders. Underlying much of the work are ideas borrowed from the neurology of Hughlings Jackson, who interpreted some symptoms as being negative in the sense that they were directly attributable to loss of function, while he regarded other phenomena as something newly produced—as positive symptoms which were released because higher integrating controls had been abolished. To give a couple of examples: in organic psychoses primitive responses, like grasp and sucking reflexes, may become re-established, or visual imagery is allowed to reach consciousness in the form of hallucinations, which may be termed "stereotyped" because they consist mainly of coloured patterns or simple animal shapes, which are described by patients coming from widely differing cultural backgrounds. In addition, Goldstein (1939) and his collaborators have sought to explain many positive symptoms of brain-damaged patients as reactions to the stress experienced by them when asked to deal with demands with which they are unable to cope. Many behaviour abnormalities in test situations, such as refusal of attempting tasks, performing substitute tasks, orderliness, stereotyped and compulsive-seeming behaviour were interpreted as means of avoiding the extreme anxiety of a "catastrophe-reaction". Disorientation, inattention and confabulation have been interpreted by other workers as attempts at minimizing immediate anxieties which arise in situations outside the psychological laboratory.

Katz *et al.* (1961) investigated the responses of recently admitted senile and arteriosclerotic dements to the stress presented by interviews and psychological tests. With the exception of a small minority who were too severely deteriorated or who had a consistently paranoid attitude, these old people showed considerable motivation towards doing well, and were co-operative and helpful in their attitudes. All the same, many of their responses were deviant in various ways and to a varying extent of severity. The mechanisms at work were conceptualised in the following fashion. (1) *Warding off* or *anticipatory control:* a patient might remark "I don't want to answer any more questions". Patients who in this and similar ways had assumed some sort of control over the situation, would then cheerfully go on to attempt all questions put to them. (2) *Time buying:* patients would use delaying tactics, exaggerate their sensory disabilities (I have yet to meet the patient who did not leave her spectacles behind before coming to an interview!), give substitute answers, launch into a diatribe on the subject, but then finally give the correct answer. (3) *Coping with failure:* failure was rarely accepted, but usually rationalised or explained away; often patients attempted to withdraw from the situation altogether. The type of response of the patient to stress was found to correspond with his level of integration. It was sometimes *situation-orientated,* i.e. the patients accepted the rules of the interview situation and implied motivation to operate within these rules. They might even acknowledge failure, but more often would have recourse to substitute responses, possibly betraying that somewhere they knew the correct answers but could only produce a near miss. A common substitute response was to start reminiscing or confabulating. Some patients appeared to misunderstand the question, exaggerating their deafness. The other type of response was *anxiety-binding*. This was less appropriate, and indicated that the situation was arousing considerable anxiety. The patient's behaviour might be socially inappropriate in that the patient did not recognise the interview situation as such but might act as the host, or become flirtatious, flattering or inappropriately anecdotal. (These may have been the kind of patients who preserve a social façade, and often deceive uninitiated doctors into assuming that they are mentally normal.) Other anxiety-binding responses were looked upon as frankly defensive: excuses such as "We never studied that at school" or "Ask my daughter, she will be able to tell"; boasting, denial "There is nothing wrong with me", or even projection, "You are trying to get me more upset with these questions". (4) *Disturbed and disruptive responses* showed themselves by outbursts of anger, weeping, withdrawal or hypochondriacal complaints. (5) *Disintegrative responses:* some patients produced delusional complaints (e.g. of maltreatment or theft by staff), illusions, hallucinations, echolalia and stereotyped movements. It is claimed that these phenomena occurred mainly under the stress of the interview, or were aggravated by it.

Patients tended to shift from one type of response to the other, depending on the amount of stress to which they felt themselves subjected. Other workers have shown that the performance of senile dements can be significantly improved by reducing stress, e.g. by giving them additional cues (Williams, 1956), and conversely that acute confusion can be produced by placing them in a dark room and depriving them in this fashion of all visual cues (Cameron, 1941).

Related to the suggestion that defence-against-anxiety mechanisms of a kind similar to those used by neurotics may be important factors in the behaviour disturbances of patients with cerebral deterioration, are views concerning the relationship between the symptomatology of dementia and previous personality. People with personality weaknesses and character defects who have earlier in life responded to stresses with minor or major psychiatric symptoms, might be expected to be especially prone to show "positive" symptoms in the course of a dementing illness in old age. Clinical studies (Post, 1944) have strengthened the impression that there are two types of both senile and arteriosclerotic dementia; one might be termed "simple" in that the clinical picture consists mainly of defects.

> Mr. C., *aet*. 85, came from a normal family, and worked his way up in life to become an elementary school teacher. By passing additional examinations at the age of 50 he finally reached the level of teaching in secondary schools. He had been happily married and was a much beloved father, easy to get on with at home, and a good mixer with many interests and hobbies. He went through a prostatectomy and the loss of his wife without psychological disturbances at the age of 75. However, since the age of 83 there had been increasing loss of memory and other symptoms of mental deterioration. His family were able to look after him, even when he began to wander away aimlessly. Finally, one week before admission, he became uncontrollably restless and experienced visual hallucinations. This was a terminal confusional state due to congestive heart failure, of which he died 6 days later.

Sometimes dementia affecting cheerful, optimistic and outgoing personalities is characterised by euphoria, restlessness, a certain amount of aggressiveness and an exaggeration of the pottering activities of elderly people, with hiding and hoarding of worthless rubbish. This condition has been termed "presbyophrenia". Dementia with more prominent psychotic symptoms, belonging to the affective or schizophrenic reaction types, is usually found in people with abnormal previous personalities. One case may be quoted:

> Mr. S., *aet*. 71, had one sister who passed through a severe depressive illness at the age of 50. He had been content to live with a brother all his life, had failed to make friends outside the family, and had never evinced any interest in the opposite sex. He was very mean, and his only hobby had been small speculations in stocks and shares. He had always been very hypochondriacal, and had accumulated a collection of over 100 homeopathic medicines. For a year before admission he had become increasingly senile, both physically and mentally. He grew quarrelsome and sought reassurance about numerous real and imagined peccadilloes of his earlier life. Finally, he developed attacks of rage and perplexity, and began to express a variety of unsystematised paranoid delusions, especially the belief that his loss of memory was brought about by violet rays and by the heat of electric wires (he was an electrician by trade). Following admission his dementia increased, his talk became incoherent, and his delusions could not be elicited any longer. At first he was irritably depressed, but later he became continuously euphoric.

Dements with ill adjusted, difficult previous personalities and with disorders of mood, behaviour and experiencing are more likely to find their way into mental hospitals than old people with lovable personalities and only "negative" symptoms of dementia. In fact, only 30 of 79 consecutive admissions for senile or arteriosclerotic dementia had normal previous personalities, and only 8 of this group with normal personalities had psychotic ("positive") symptoms in addition to dementia (Post, 1944). Among abnormal personality traits, rigidity and obsessional trends or characters were especially prominent. Recently, Oakley (1962) confirmed that senile and arteriosclerotic dements in a mental hospital scored significantly higher on obsessional personality ratings than a matched control group of mentally healthy old people.

AETIOLOGY

In recent years it has become fashionable to stress the significance of dynamic personality factors in the causation of the organic psychoses of old age, and to play down the importance of cerebral pathology. This movement derived from Gruenthal's (1927) investigations. Though he found that by and large there was positive correlation between degree of senile deterioration and severity of neuropathological changes, he had to admit, like others since him, that there were a number of subjects where brains had shown atrophy and various senile changes who had not suffered any clinically recognized dementia. He therefore suggested that senile changes and cerebral atrophy occurring in an old person were not sufficient causes of senile dementia, but that another, as yet unidentified, pathogenic factor had to be present as well. Rothschild (1937, 1942) asserted that in his own material of senile and arteriosclerotic cases, there was only a very crude relationship between macroscopic as well as histological abnormalities and intellectual changes. He strongly suggested that severity of dementia was not related to the extent of cerebral damage, but to the different ways in which people were able to compensate for it.

> "In other words, patients with senile or arteriosclerotic psychoses should not be regarded merely as passive carriers of a morbid anatomic process. One should attempt to estimate to what extent more personal factors are concerned in each case. In many cases, such a study suggests that the qualities of the living person and his life experiences are the most important factors in the origin of the mental breakdown. . . . Thus, there emerges a more meaningful picture of the psychosis as an end state in a long process which has its roots not just in certain impersonal tissue alterations but in psychological stresses and in social problems which affect the ageing population".
>
> (Rothschild, 1956.)

These views, which were consonant with a more hopeful outlook in geriatrics, have had considerable influence on psychiatric thought. However, Williams *et al.* (1942) pointed out that there were striking differences in the previous personalities and life records of patients with arteriosclerotic and senile dementia, respectively. Their arteriosclerotics were, as a group, well-adjusted socially and domestically, while most of their seniles had become socially deteriorated or isolated. They concluded that senile dementia developed in the wake of long-standing social deterioration, which was mainly the result of earlier personality defects, whereas cerebralarteriosclerotic damage was a physiogenic event, relatively independent of personality or environmental factors.

Closer analysis of Rothschild's findings has shown that he over-emphasised the occasional case where there had been serious disagreement between clinical assessment and severity of anatomical changes. Corsellis (1962) pointed out that discrepancies between Rothschild's clinical and pathological ratings on a five-point scale were rarely larger than one point. In his own study, Corsellis demonstrated conclusively that there existed a strong positive correlation between a clinical diagnosis of arteriosclerotic or of senile dementia and the severity of independently assessed brain changes. The brains of patients with organic psychoses were rated as more severely affected by vascular changes, atrophy, neurofibrillary changes and formation of senile plaques, than the brains of patients with a diagnosis of affective, schizophrenic or paranoid illness. These differences were in most instances statistically highly significant, and occurred over and above an increase of pathological features, both in organic and in functional psychotics, with rising age alone. Again, there were a few functional cases with marked cerebral changes, and some patients diagnosed during life as suffering from dementia, but showing only slight macroscopic and microscopic vascular or parenchymal abnormalities in the brain.

To what extent is senility the terminal phase of a lifelong faulty personality development, or the result of impersonal factors, described in question-begging fashion as "abnormal ageing of the brain"? Attempts at solving this problem can probably not be pushed much further with present-day, or even future, methods of investigation. Perhaps the question, based as it is on a dualistic body–mind concept, is misconceived. At present, all we can say is that mental senility and physical deterioration of the brain tend to parallel one another. In addition, it should be remembered that investigations of dementia in old age have been largely confined to patients admitted to mental hospitals, either because nobody was willing to look after them any longer or because they had become aggressive, depressed or severely deluded. Patients of either kind are likely to have had difficult and deviant personalities, and senile dements coming under psychiatric care may be an unrepresentative sample of persons affected with this disorder.

As many dements enter hospital for social and personality reasons, or only on account of psychotic symptoms, it has been suggested that in the majority of cases, dementia in old age (especially of the senile type) is not an illness at all but merely an exaggeration and acceleration of a statistically normal process. In support, it may be pointed out that, not infrequently, old people become confused and present a psychiatric problem for the first time after the death of their spouse, moving away of children or changes of home. In many instances this breakdown turns out to be not just an acute confusional state but a phase in a dementing process, which on closer inquiry is found to have been going on for some time. Sudden removal of social support had precipitated more acute symptoms, and the suggestion arises that "we all dement provided we live long enough", but that the appearance of an overt disturbance calling for psychiatric intervention depends on other factors such as physical illnesses, difficult personalities, disunited families, bereavements or sudden social upheavals.

A number of studies have confirmed that there are many more dements in the community than are ever admitted to hospital, presumably because they are adequately cared for and protected by their families and friends. In New York State (Survey of Mental Health Research Unit, 1960/61) 6·3 per cent of people over 65 living in their own homes "had enough manifest symptoms of the psychoses of ageing to be judged to be unable to care for themselves or to be a danger to themselves or others, according to the prevailing practices in implementing the provisions of the New York State laws regarding involuntary certification of patients to mental hospitals". This proportion rose from 3·2 per cent for ages 65–69 to 30·1 per cent among persons aged 85 and over. Of interest in the present context is the corollary: that even over the age of 85, 69·9 per cent of people were still able to care for themselves and were in no way a danger to themselves and others. Other investigations have confirmed that, even among people reaching the highest age levels, only a proportion are demented. There are, moreover, sex differences. Parsons (1962) in his survey of old people in their own homes, found significant memory impairment, which was not necessarily associated with generalised dementia, in over half of women over 80, but much less frequently in men surviving to this age. Above the age of 85, 86 per cent of women were reported by their friends as having suffered deterioration of various personality facets, such as interests, ability to plan ahead, proneness to anxiety, irritability, etc. Only 67 per cent of men over 85 had shown this kind of deterioration.

Numerous surveys have indicated that men tend to die earlier than women, but that when they do survive they remain healthier, mentally and physically. Like other defects, which manifest themselves in old age, senile dementia shows the phenomenon of sex-linkage, suggesting a genetic basis. The view that this disorder is a circumscribed disease and does not just present one extreme of the distribution of mental age changes in the population, is also strengthened by the frequently attested occurrence of a positive family history for late life dementia in excess of "expectation" among patients with this disorder and with pre-senile dementia (for details see Kallmann, 1957; Sjoegren et al., 1952; Larsson et al., 1963).

In addition, psychological and psychophysiological workers have shown a number of ways in which demented old people differ from subjects who have aged normally. Grewell (1953) pointed out that a woman of 84 might not be as spry as one of 20; that she might be forgetful and not always able to give the correct date. She might well show patchiness of test scores, most likely a lowering on performance as against verbal and vocabulary items, but, compared with a patient suffering from senile dementia she would clearly be a rational and well-preserved person, taking an interest in events in her sphere of life, a pride in her appearance, and having a sympathetic attitude towards her neighbours. More recently, Kral (1962) stressed that there were two types of memory dysfunction in old people. In the "benign" type there is inability to recall relatively unimportant data and parts of an experience (like a name, a place or a date), whereas the experience itself, of which the forgotten items form a part, can be recalled. Furthermore, matters which are not available for recollection on one occasion, may be recalled at another time. In the "malignant" type there is, in addition, inability to recall events in the recent past, and not just relatively unimportant items or parts of an experience; the experience as such cannot be recalled at all. Confabulation may be resorted to, and the condition is, in fact, identical with a senile Korsakoff syndrome; it presents as part and parcel of a dementia due to senile brain degeneration. Like others, Kral found that subjects with the malignant type of memory disorder were physically less fit than those with benign memory difficulties, and that their mortality rate was significantly higher. Significantly shorter survival was one of the characteristics of elderly psychiatric patients whose memory disorders lay largely in a failure to learn and recall new material (Sanderson and Inglis, 1961). Dorken (1958) pointed out that the orderly relationship between the decline of various mental abilities and increasing age found in elderly persons no longer held in cases of senile dementia, where many younger patients with this disorder may have much lower test scores than some older cases. He agreed with Botwinnick and Birren (1951), who found that scores on various sub-tests declined to a differing extent in normal aged subjects as compared with dements. They concluded from these qualitative as well as quantitative differences in declines, that dementia was entirely different from normal age deficit. Finally, senile dements fail to learn even at the simplest level, in that they are found unable to form new conditional (avoidance) reflexes (Brown *et al.*, 1961).

From the physiological angle, recent studies of cerebral oxygen uptake have also shown that patients with dementia can be sharply differentiated from normal aged subjects whose average values were only 9 per cent below the level of young adult subjects. Severely demented old people had the lowest values of cerebral oxygen uptake, some 40 per cent below young normals, while patients with less severe mental defects had more moderate reductions—about 20 per cent (Lassen *et al.*, 1960, who summarise previous work and refer to more speculative findings).

THERAPEUTIC CONSIDERATIONS

The traditional arrangement, by which the description of an illness is followed by a full account of its treatment, has been abandoned in this book because most elderly psychiatric patients suffer at the same time from several disorders. For the sake of clarity, illnesses have to be described as separate entities, but in practice we usually have to treat the patient for a number of different illnesses at the same time. To avoid reduplications and repetition, I propose to give a full account of current methods of management and treatment, with indications of their employment, separately in a special final chapter. Theoretical and general therapeutic and prognostic consideration will, however, be mentioned at the end of each section.

The therapeutic approach is relatively straightforward in acute senile confusional states, but only because in most cases a medical or surgical diagnosis can be made, and the therapeutic problem converted from a psychiatric into a somatic one. Turning to the chronic confusional states (chronic brain syndromes), i.e. the dementias of old age, their basic causes are by many held to be somatic also. The treatment of arteriosclerotic dementia may then be regarded essentially as the prevention and treatment of athero-sclerosis, hypertension or renal disease. In the case of senile dementia, treatment ought to be directed towards as yet only suspected pathogenic factors—biochemical ones—at a guess.

In the absence of any real and fundamental knowledge, numerous treatments have been introduced at one time or another for patients with chronic brain syndromes. They have all been due to hunches derived from clinical impressions and more or less related research findings. Many successful and established treatments in general medicine and in psychiatry have originated in this way, but as far as the dementias of old age are concerned there are no therapies which have become generally accepted. This is true, even of the few which were introduced after controlled trials had shown beneficial effects in the original samples of patients, e.g. monosodium L-glutamate has not become a universally accepted remedy, though favourable reports have been appearing since 1955 (Gasster, 1961). This disappointing state of affairs was revealed fairly recently (Post, 1959), and there is no need to review in detail past therapeutic investigations, especially those referring to the use of vitamins and hormones. A few points may be taken up because they relate to more recent research findings.

In spite of early promise, inhalations of oxygen and administrations of respiratory enzymes have not become established treatments of senile dementia. This is hardly surprising, since their rationale, diminished cerebral oxygen uptake in senile dementia, is almost certainly due to the diminution in the number of living brain cells.

More relevant may be the claim advanced by Wahal and Riggs (1960) that parenchymatous brain changes found in younger patients, who had died in congestive heart failure, were identical with those seen in the dementias of old age. The effective treatment of cardiac insufficiencies in elderly people may well prove important in preventing or delaying the onset of mental deterioration.

One of the most recent claims to successful treatment of memory disorders concerns the use of ribonucleic acid (RNA) (Cameron and Solyom, 1961; Cameron et al., 1962). The rationale of this treatment appears to have changed since experimentation began. Originally (Cameron, 1958), the therapy was introduced because RNA was known to play a leading role in the process of protein synthesis which goes on continually in nerve cells. Buerger (1958) had in fact shown that the amount of RNA in human brains declined in old age (while that of DNA increased). Later on came the discovery that the effects of mutation, of synthesis of new antibodies, and of other newly "learnt" adaptation mechanisms, were encoded in the molecular structure of certain nucleic acids, including RNA, and the suggestion was made that in this way fresh "information" was preserved and passed on to later generations of cells. Dingman and Sporn (1961) pointed out that one was dealing here with an example of physiological learning and memory. They suggested that psychological memory traces in the CNS were produced by altering the arrangements of RNA molecules, and they produced experimental evidence in support of this hypothesis. After oral trials, Cameron and his group of collaborators developed a technique by which large quantities of RNA could be administered intravenously to arteriosclerotic and senile dements. Test results before and after treatment (with tests whose practice effects are not quoted!), as well as reports of nurses and relatives, suggested that there was a significant improvement of memory function, especially in less severely demented subjects. This form of treatment, which is based on a somewhat audacious analogy between physiological and psychological learning, is still very much at the experimental stage.

Possibilities of treating senile deterioration have also been explored from the psychosocial angle. While accepting a cerebral basis for senile dementia, the important contributions to the actual disabilities stemming from personality and social factors have been rightly stressed. Numerous investigations have demonstrated that deteriorated old people in the community and demented patients in hospital belong to the lower socio-economic groups, have never married, or have been widowed, to a significantly greater extent than their normal contemporaries. It may be held that people fail to rise socially, or decline in status during life, because they are poorly endowed intellectually, and that persons of low intelligence tend to dement prematurely. This has in fact been demonstrated for mongoloid imbeciles (Jelgersma, 1958). People who fail to get married have frequently been shown as unduly prone to all kinds of psychiatric disturbances. But, no constitutional factors can possibly explain the excessively high frequency of dementia (making allowance for age) among widowed persons. It has, therefore, been suggested that lack of social contacts and of opportunities to keep up interests and skills may hasten or even precipitate senile dementia.

This hypothesis was tested experimentally (Cosin et al., 1958). We found that a variety of simple occupations and of social activities were capable of improving the general level of behaviour in senile dements, but that the beneficial effects of these measures evaporated rapidly. Moreover, our subjects failed to resume any kind of initiative, as if they had lost for good the capacity of self-motivation. In comparison with a control group, the subjects of the experiment did not show any significant slowing of mental decline over a period of 6–12 months. Possibly, better results might be obtained with psychological, and indeed with any measures, if they could be applied to less severely deteriorated patients. I have previously speculated (Post, 1958) on the generally experienced difficulty of discovering persons in the early stages of dementia, when treatment might be more successful as only few changes have become irreversible. Do relatives and family doctors fail to observe early mental decline? Are their attitudes too fatalistic, or does dementia in fact manifest itself relatively suddenly, and only when previously ignored decline reaches a certain threshold?

In concluding this chapter I have to admit regretfully that as yet there are no effective and proven treatments of the dementias of old age. Considerable amelioration can, however, be effected by correct management, a subject to which we shall return in the final chapter, devoted to treatment.

CHAPTER IV

AFFECTIVE DISORDERS

THE IMPORTANCE OF MOOD DISORDERS IN OLD AGE

It is impossible to overestimate the extent to which disorders of mood affect mental health adversely. Among Western peoples, anxiety and depression are much more commonly encountered than elation, excitement or exaltation, and mild anxious-depressive disorders are often the real reasons for which so many people consult their doctors with minor physical complaints.

The ease with which people become tense or depressed varies with age. Adolescence and early adult life are well recognised stormy periods, and questionnaire studies suggest that people between the ages of 30 and 50 show the greatest emotional stability. After that age, mood tends to become increasingly labile. Crabbedness, surliness, dejection and discontent have long been regarded as attributes of senility, and the great frequency of mild mood disturbances in the elderly has been confirmed by recent field studies. This increase with age of mild affective disturbances is paralleled by a rising incidence of more severe depressive mental disorders, as reflected in hospital admissions and suicide rates.

Basing herself on first admissions to three mental hospitals in the London area, Norris (1959) estimated the rates for first admissions on account of manic-depressive psychoses and involutional melancholia at different ages. The frequency at which affective illnesses requiring admission first manifested themselves in women rose only slightly between the ages of 20 and 35 (from 120 to 250 per million of each age group), but from then on steadily to about 470 per million between the ages of 60 and 65. In men, first admission rates ran at about half the level of that of women, but rose steeply after the age of 40 to about 375 per million of men between the ages of 55 and 60. First admissions dropped sharply during old age, but by the age of 75 there were still some 100 men per million who were admitted for the first time in life with affective disorders. By contrast, a diagnosis of these conditions was made much more rarely (*ca.* 25 per million) for the first time in women over 75.

The overall incidence of suicide and the relationship between suicide and age vary from culture to culture. In pre-war China suicide among the elderly is said to have been low, allegedly on account of the favoured position of the aged. In Japan suicide is alleged to be the commonest cause of death among the young. In Britain suicide rates of both sexes increase strikingly with age. Sainsbury (1962) found that a sharp rise began in the fifth decade of life, and that it was more marked as well as more sustained into late life in men (rising to about 420 per million in them as against to 150 per million in women). Successful or attempted suicide of the elderly tended to be preceded by depression of some duration in from 50 to 70 per cent of cases, while in younger persons suicidal acts were much more frequently explosive responses of unstable personalities to immediate life stresses. "Crises in personal relationships, in particular marital and family quarrels, precipitate suicide most often in the young, less in the middle, and least in the old age group." Emotional social isolation, bereavement and physical ill health were important factors of suicide among the aged, and the high suicide rate in old men might be due to retirement affecting them more severely than women. Furthermore, suicides tended to decrease after 65 in men belonging to the higher social classes, but increased in men of lower social status, presumably because they retired in less secure economic circumstances or had fewer opportunities for varied interests and outlets.

Enough has been said to show why the recognition and treatment of affective disorders ought to be among the main concerns of physicians and psychiatrists practising among elderly people: (1) depressive disorders manifest themselves most frequently late in life, (2) suicidal tendencies increase with age to a frightening extent.

MILD MOOD DISORDERS

Among the elderly there is a marked trend towards developing anxiety and feelings of hopelessness of a milder type. A research team in North Carolina (Busse *et al.*, 1955) reported the occurrence of depressive mood changes in 48 per cent of persons over 60 who were unable to work, attending an out-patient clinic for various physical disorders, and suffering financial hardships. Depressive spells occurred in an only slightly smaller proportion of persons (44 per cent) who were retired, but in good health and economic circumstances. Depressions were reported by a smaller, but still sizeable, proportion (25 per cent) of old people able to continue in some type of work, possibly because occupation warded off depression, or because the kind of people who continue to work beyond the age of retirement also tend to show less severe temperamental changes with ageing. Most people denied that they had suffered depressive spells of similar frequency or duration earlier in life. After the age of 60 they experienced affective disturbances about once a month, lasting from a few hours to a few days, and during them they were so discouraged, worried or troubled that they would often feel that there was no reason to go on living. They frequently wished for a painless death, but only one subject of the investigation admitted to ever having made a suicidal attempt. They were often aware of some precipitating experience, and as feelings of guilt and self-reproach were absent, the investigators concluded that they were dealing with reactive rather than so-called endogenous depressions. In fact, none of these subjects was admitted under psychiatric care during several years of subsequent observation. The treatment of these mild mood disturbances falls entirely within the scope of the family doctor, and psychiatrists have too little experience in the management of these allegedly very frequent problems to give an authoritative account. I have to limit myself to discussing recognition, classification and outlook of the more definite and more severe affective illnesses occurring in old people.

MANIA

Only between 5 and 10 per cent of elderly people referred for the treatment of affective disorders exhibit the excited or elated phase. While the recognition of depression may be long delayed because the disorder so often occurs in habitually morose, hypochondriacal and self-concerned old people, an eruption of excessive activity, of over-energetic behaviour, and of expansive over-talkativeness in the life of a quietly retired old man is unlikely to remain unnoticed for long. Even when the disorder occurs in a normally cheerful, active, domineering and irascible old man, repercussions on the environment are so severe that medical aid is soon sought.

Mania in the elderly differs in some respects from that seen in younger people, and differentiation from other excited states may present problems. This may best be illustrated by referring to the case records of a patient who was observed in four attacks and where initial diagnostic doubts were eventually resolved completely.

This man of 75 had retired 10 years previously from the lower grades of the Civil Service. He had a family history of depressive illnesses and alcoholism, but had never been ill himself. Eight years earlier he had passed through a brief period when his alcoholic intake had been causing concern; at other times he had been a moderate drinker, extroverted, always optimistic and cheerful, with many outside interests. The only abnormal trait was his jealousy; he had always objected to his wife having conversations with other men. His marriage had, however, been sexually satisfactory, and intercourse had only ceased 5 months before his first admission, after he had been ill with a protracted attack of bronchitis. On recovery he began to work feverishly, but somewhat haphazardly, in house and garden. He ate well, but lost weight and sleep. He began to accuse his wife (aged 70) of having sexual relations with a nephew (a bachelor, aged 50), who had been lodging at their home for some time. As he began to make violent scenes, and threatened to strangle them both, he was compulsorily removed to a mental observation ward, and later transferred to our unit.

He exhibited a number of typical manic features. He claimed to be able to make large sums on the turf. He proposed to give the money away for charitable purposes, including a sizeable donation to the hospital. Numerous written criticisms and orders were issued to the nursing staff, towards whom he behaved alternately in an imperious and flirtatious manner. In a letter to his wife he boasted: ". . . am feeling full of beans, etc., etc., have just dated two lovely girls, one for the pictures (Sat) (dark) *Spanish*, the other *not quite certain where we shall* go, but probably in the country somewhere where it is somewhat *seclouded* [*sic*] for tea, she is *Brunette* of *course* my *special colour*, & boy what a *smasher*, good old english. Now about this hospital business. . . ."

There were, however, the following atypical points:

(1) Though claiming to be happy, the patient usually looked tense, drawn and miserable.

(2) He was over-talkative, but his talk was repetitive and usually anecdotal. There was little flight of association (never more

marked than in above quotation), but rather a circumstantial meandering with eventual return to the subject.

(3) He firmly believed that his wife was unfaithful to him with the nephew, and persisted in relating how he had caught them in suggestive situations, how he had discovered the usual tell-tale stains on the bed linen, etc.

(4) He looked bewildered, and consistently made mistakes about dates and about the sequence of events preceding admission. His arithmetic was poor, and he thought the 1939 war had lasted from 1947 to 1956 (the year of the first admission).

As so often with elderly manics, these symptoms and signs suggested that the patient's excited state might be due to a pathological cerebral process. A combination of euphoria, over-activity and intellectual impairment is described in a type of senile dementia, which in the past has been labelled "presbyophrenia"; but in this condition persistent paranoid delusions are not seen. They are, of course, the main feature of the paranoid form of senile dementia, especially ridiculous delusions of sexual jealousy. A similar combination is encountered in some alcoholic psychoses. Finally, paranoid schizophrenia in the elderly is often monosymptomatic, and is sometimes triggered off psychologically, possibly, on the basis of a jealous personality, by impotence and the presence of a younger man.

On further study, the duration of symptoms and non-fluctuating preservation of full awareness excluded the diagnosis of an acute senile confusional state. Neurological examination and investigations produced no localising signs (of arteriosclerotic foci or of a tumour), and excluded G.P.I. The fact that a short course of treatment with chlorpromazine terminated the excitement did not negate the possibility of gradual senile mental changes being the basic cause of the psychosis. However, this possibility was excluded over the subsequent five years by the fact that the patient did not ever again show memory difficulties, and that his abilities did not decline. Formal psychological testing confirmed this. Recent and continuing alcoholism could also be excluded. A diagnosis of senile paranoid schizophrenia was more difficult to demolish, as the patient did not gain retrospective "insight". For a long time he continued to believe that his wife had had an affair with the nephew, but had repented of her conduct. In his second breakdown he was convinced that the affair had been resumed, though by then the nephew was no longer living in his house. In the third attack there were no delusions of jealousy, but he believed that a neighbour had been raiding his vegetable plot and had been stealing his choicest carrots. In the fourth and, up to date, last illness, there was no paranoid content at all; moreover, on recovery he pooh-poohed his past ideas concerning his wife and nephew as "nonsense". In the meantime, he had resumed regular marital sexual intercourse, and his initial loss of libido had clearly been a symptom rather than a cause of his illness.

Many elderly manics exhibit even more atypical features than the patient whose case we have just quoted. Their surliness, irritability and lack of infectious gaiety, together with ludicrous paranoid sexual ideas or delusions of theft have in the past been attributed to the pathoplastic effects of mental senility. It is true that flight of ideas, so notable in the talk of young manics, is frequently replaced by senile anecdotal and circumstantial garrulity, but in other respects, atypical features in senile manics are more convincingly explained by the presence of depressive admixtures. Mixed states in younger patients are often misdiagnosed because the simultaneous presence of manic and melancholic mood disorders tends to produce perplexity with disorientation, together with paranoid ways of experiencing; "organic confusional state" or "acute schizophrenic episode" are frequent initial diagnoses. In elderly manics some depression is almost always present at the same time. In our case it was noted that the patient looked tense, drawn and miserable though claiming that he felt very happy. During his first attack he showed some disorientation and memory disturbance, and we shall presently see that the sudden onset of depression in elderly people is quite commonly associated with temporary intellectual impairment. Also, our patient's paranoid delusions did not reflect increased self-esteem, as seen in pure mania, but centred around the depressive theme of loss; at first loss of his marital honour, and later, from the sublime to the ridiculous, of his best carrots.

DEPRESSION

Diagnostic difficulties arise in practice in a small proportion of cases, if only because so often similar depressive episodes have occurred earlier in life. The affective nature of a disorder is likely to remain unrecognised when it is mild, without any obvious changes in appearance or behaviour, and when it presents as an exacerbation of long-standing anxious, hypochondriacal, phobic or obsessional propensities. Patients of this sort are frequently regarded as chronic neurotics, who are finally becoming senile, until they make suicidal attempts or are referred in desperation to psychiatrists, because their demands and complaints are wearing down their friends. At the other extreme, severely disordered patients, who appear confused and inaccessible, may be wrongly diagnosed as suffering from arterio-sclerotic or senile dementia. Finally, in the presence of marked persecutory symptoms, a diagnosis of depression may not be entertained, and the patients may be looked upon as senile para-phrenics or dements with a paranoid symptomatology. Before we run the risk of losing ourselves in details of description, differentiation and classification, I am anxious to make one point; it cannot be emphasised too strongly that anxiety and depression themselves, as well as the symptoms derived from them, are very unpleasant and cause considerable suffering. Especially in the case of elderly people, affective symptoms tend to respond quickly to a variety of modern therapeutic measures, and these should not be withheld on account of unresolved diagnostic difficulties. It may be objected quite correctly that in many cases relief of symptoms may be incomplete and only very temporary, especially when the affective disturbance has occurred in the setting of progressive physical disease, most commonly cerebral arteriosclerosis. However, we shall see that attempts to assign the true significance of many features in the clinical pictures presented by elderly depressives are fraught with uncertainties. In the past there has been a tendency to overvalue the importance of various phenomena suggesting cerebral disorders and deterioration. I shall leave it to the reader to decide to what extent ominous head-shakings may not have been due to the wish on the part of specialists to be absolved from further dealings with these troublesome and not very attractive patients.

A more detailed discussion of depressive illness in old age is only possible by describing the varied clinical pictures under a number of descriptive headings. In doing this we are not proposing yet another system of classifications, but our sub-types are so many Aunt Sallies, put up only in order to be knocked down promptly.

1. ORGANIC DEPRESSIONS

Depressive symptoms not infrequently occur in patients suffering from cerebral disease. The literature contains many references to cerebral tumours presenting as depressions, but among the elderly the association between depression and cerebral arteriosclerosis or, to a lesser extent, senile cerebral deterioration is overwhelmingly more common. The following case record will illustrate how depression may sometimes appear in an organic setting:

> Mr. R., aged 73, a shopkeeper, was admitted because for the preceding week or two he had been depressed, quiet and deluded in thinking that he owed large sums of money in taxes. He had begun to talk of suicide, to eat poorly, and to sleep badly. He was referred for admission because he had become helpless and unable to find his way about in his own home. In hospital he was agitated and miserable; he believed that he owed £800, and imagined various business difficulties. At times he was correctly orientated, had a full grasp of events of personal and general significance, but at other times he made numerous mistakes and tended to lose his way around the ward. There was no neurological abnormality, but his blood pressure varied between 120/80 and 160/100 mm Hg.

The patient's daughter and one of his brothers had suffered from depressive illnesses, and the patient himself had suffered a previous attack some six years earlier. In spite of the absence of neurological findings, the presence of a pathological cerebral process was strongly suspected because on inquiry it emerged that his earlier depression had some rather odd features; he had been not only depressed, but had also claimed that money had been stolen from the till. The money was eventually found hidden all over the house, and this hiding of objects and claiming them to be stolen is a well-known behaviour disorder of elderly dements. The patient recovered after a few weeks, but was never again entrusted with money matters.

> During his second depression the patient scored like a person with brain damage on a number of learning tests, and a pneumoencephalogram suggested the presence of generalised cerebral atrophy. Like some of the brain-damaged patients, he responded to imipramine by becoming unmistakably confused and disorientated. On discontinuing the drug, this disturbance cleared, and so did his depressive symptoms. Learning tests gave normal results, and clinically he performed tasks of memory and orientation invariably well.
>
> He remained mildly dejected following discharge, and from time to time expressed hypochondriacal fears. After six months he suddenly became confused, and at night would imagine himself in his shop removing imaginary merchandise from imaginary shelves (i.e. showing occupational delirium). He again believed that thefts were occurring. On re-admission the affect

accompanying his talk about poverty and debts seemed shallow, and at times even euphoric. His performance on tests was consistently lower than during the first admission, and he was variably disorientated. In addition, tremor, apraxia and astereognosis were noted in his left upper limb.

It is suggested that this patient's illness is best understood as a series of subacute confusional states due to an intermittent pathological process in the brain; localising signs began to appear in the third attack, and a cerebrovascular disorder seemed the most likely diagnosis. Apart from "organic" symptoms like confusion, hoarding, and delusions of theft, the patient showed initially well-defined melancholic symptoms, presumably on account of an inherited constitutional disposition to the affective reaction type, which for the first time in his life became mobilised during organic-confusional episodes.

More commonly one finds patients with recurrent affective illnesses on the background of a slowly progressive dementing process. Probably the commonest association between cerebral disease and depression is exemplified by this case of depression following upon a cerebral incident.

Mr. M., a retired solicitor's clerk, was discharged from the army during the 1914 war with "shell shock"; on inquiry the symptoms had consisted of anxiety, hypochondriasis and financial preoccupations of delusional severity. At the age of 60 he had been depressed, talking of suicide, but recovering after a few weeks in a general hospital. Aged 72, after a prodromal period of carelessness and forgetfulness, he suddenly developed a right-sided homonymous hemianopia. Within a few weeks he became gloomy and morose as well as unduly worried over his financial affairs. He developed a fear that he might kill his wife. He had always had marked obsessional personality traits, but the fear during this illness was not just a phobia, because one night his wife woke with the patient's hands round her neck. This led to his admission, the patient recovering from his depression after a few weeks of psychotherapeutic management.

The patient was followed over the subsequent ten years. He did not dement, but developed diabetes, and had an episode when he was unable to hold a pencil, and was reported as having exhibited transitory pyramidal signs in his right upper extremity. At that time he had again been somewhat irritable with his wife.

"Organic depression" used to be regarded as a special syndrome characterised by a shallow, labile and variable affect as well as by ridiculous and ill-structured delusional preoccupations. The depression was looked upon as a passing phase during the dementing process, which was suspected of implicating parts of the brain controlling affect. However, it has become increasingly recognised that in spite of the presence of brain damage, these depressions can be very severe, with suicide not at all uncommon, and that the patient's thought-content may be indistinguishable from that seen in other elderly melancholics. Earlier workers showed that cerebral arteriosclerotics with depression usually had histories of affective illnesses earlier in life, and more recently I found that "organic" depressives had a positive family history, especially of severe affective illnesses, even more often than elderly depressives without brain damage. In addition, the follow-up studies of several workers (Kay *et al.*, 1955; Kay, 1959; Post, 1962) have conclusively demonstrated that elderly depressives do not develop over the subsequent years of their life cerebral degeneration any more frequently than elderly people in general, and considerable doubt has been thrown on the validity of the concept of "prodromal depression" or of a "neuras-thenic stage" in cerebral arteriosclerotic, senile or pre-senile dementia.

For all these reasons we are nowadays inclined to explain the occurrence of depression and dementia in the same patient by evoking coincidence or precipitation. Depression and dementia are both common disorders in old age, and their occasional occurrence in the same person is not surprising. This explanation is particularly satisfying when affective episodes recur on the background of a slowly progressive dementing process. When cerebral incidents and depres-sive symptoms occur at about the same time, it seems reasonable to assume that the cerebral disturbance mobilised the affective reaction type to which the patient was predisposed. Many physical illnesses have been found to figure in the aetiology of depressive illnesses in the elderly, but cerebrovascular disorders appear to be unduly frequent precipitants, suggesting that there is a long-suspected constitutional link between the tendency to develop vascular degeneration, on the one hand, and affective illness, on the other. We are not in a position to decide whether precipitation of depression occurs along somatic channels, or whether, at a more psycho-physiological level, the arousal of anxiety sets in motion the "depressive process" in certain people.

2. DEPRESSIVE PSEUDO-DEMENTIA

Depressed patients, especially when they are also severely perplexed, sometimes give the impression that they are impaired in awareness and disorientated (i.e. organically confused), as well as having a defective memory. They may show the "syndrome of approximate answers", and as they do not develop a dementia following recovery from the depression, the abnormality is sometimes referred to as "pseudo-dementia".

> Mr. Ch., a retired schoolmaster, had had a first depressive illness at the age of 63, recovering with ECT. Aged 69, he had to be readmitted with a six weeks' history of increasing agitation. He was very restless and apprehensive, looked perplexed and miserable, and believed that a cancer was closing up his throat. He also thought that the police were about to arrest him for some trivial sexual misdemeanour in his youth. There were no physical abnormalities, but the patient appeared to be organically confused; he did not know the name of the hospital, thought it was situated near Edenbridge instead of Eden Park, and that he had been previously admitted one year ago. He gave the year (1950) variously as 1918, 1935 and 1952. He failed to learn his psychiatrist's name. In addition he telescoped the dates of various events in his life, placed the first war correctly, but was unable to give the dates of the 1939 war, and thought MacDonald had preceded Churchill as Prime Minister. These failures were not due to lack of co-operation, as he was consistently able to repeat correctly eight digits forwards and six backwards, and as he also gave excellent immediate renderings of a brief story.
> He recovered after four ECTs, and a week or two later his performance on tests of memory function was in keeping with educational background and almost faultless. He continued to enjoy his retirement, but at the age of 73 had to be admitted once again on account of agitation and a fear that he had a growth in his neck. Cognitive impairment was noted again, clearing together with the agitated depression after five ECTs.

It is of interest to note that in both admissions the Wechsler Bellevue Intelligence Test was administered before and after successful treatment. There was no decline over the years, but on each occasion the score before treatment was lower than that after treatment. It should be pointed out that in pseudo-dementia occurring in the setting of a variety of psychiatric disorders, psychological tests often appear to indicate the presence of organic intellectual impairment, and are not useful in differentiating pseudo-dementia from real dementia. On reflection, this ought not really to be surprising, as all that psychological cognitive testing does is to examine clinical features in a more standardised and calibrated form. In fact, a current investigation is going to demonstrate that severely depressed and perplexed elderly patients, even when not showing any striking clinical signs of confusion, tend to score like organic mental patients on tests of learning new material, with the scores rising to normal levels after successful treatment. It is thus not uncommon for severe depressions to produce temporary intellectual impairment. One of the chief characteristics of these illnesses is to affect the total

4

organism, and in the elderly this often takes the form of making the patient look older, in that he assumes a shuffling gait, a coarse tremor and various rigidities. In 27 per cent of elderly depressives, abnormalities of gait, rigidities, tremors and other dubious neurological findings were discovered; in 41 per cent slight memory difficulties were noted. Over the subsequent six years these patients with dubious signs of cerebral involvement fared no worse than the rest of the cases as far as their depressions were concerned. The presence of neurological signs of doubtful significance or of slight memory difficulties did not differentiate those few patients who later on developed definite senile or arteriosclerotic disorders (Post, 1962). Isolated or doubtful neurological findings and slight cognitive defects may therefore be ignored in depressive states, as they will be evidence of early dementia in a very small proportion of cases. It may be impossible to differentiate between pseudo-dementia and a true organic confusional state, though two observations help to exclude the presence of a dementing process: (1) the history suggests strongly that up to the appearance of depressive symptoms there had been no decline of abilities and memory; (2) in contrast to organically confused patients, there is no attempt to confabulate or to make facile excuses for not knowing answers, but instead there is a tendency for the patient to counter (perhaps negativistically) all questions by "I don't know".

For immediate clinical purposes there is now a tendency to pay less attention to whether or not depressions are "functional" or "organic", as they tend to respond equally well to treatment as far as immediate removal of symptoms is concerned. In the presence of definite neurological signs and/or organic mental symptoms, it is clearly desirable to attempt to rule out by investigations (as far as is permitted by the patient's mental state and behaviour) the presence of treatable intracranial diseases, especially tumours or GPI. But if these can be reasonably excluded, the presence of definite dementia, pseudo-dementia or "early dementia" should not interfere with the determined treatment of depression.

3. SENILE MELANCHOLIA

This label has in the past been attached to a group of depressives falling ill for the first time in their eighth or ninth decades with psychopathologically very colourful symptoms. Motor-agitation is usually severe, but the depressive affect seems shallow or, at any rate, is poorly communicated. Instead, there are severe hypochondriacal delusions and convictions of tremendous guilt. Moreover, the hypochondriasis is bizarre: old women, though intellectually well preserved, may believe themselves pregnant, and may speak of having committed "the unforgivable sin". Their expressions of guilt have a grandiose flavour: "the worst person that ever lived", "will not be allowed to die but roam about as a disembodied spirit". Self-accusations of this sort may well have led to the stake a few centuries ago; one of these modern witches misinterpreted distant noises as "atom bombs being exploded through my wickedness". Related to these delusions of enormity, are nihilistic ideas concerning the contents of the body, Cotard's *délire de négation*. "My stomach has gone", "food drops from my chest into my belly", "my lungs have rotted away", "my bones are all hollow", "my head is empty", "my brain is shrunk and lies at the bottom of my skull", "my head is filled with rice pudding". More frequently these ideas are expressed in an equally nihilistic but more sophisticated fashion, i.e. a man attributing an inability to open his bowels to atrophy of their muscular coat. It used to be thought that these patients' illnesses invariably pursued a chronic course ending in senile dementia. Though much space is given to the description of this disorder in textbooks, nowadays it is only rarely seen, possibly because many more patients with less severe illnesses are admitted to psychiatric hospitals. One case will suffice to illustrate the symptomatology of this type of depression, as well as the unsatisfactory course often taken after electroconvulsive therapy.

Mr. Co., aged 75, had been a widower for some twenty years. He had always been strict and uncompromising in his outlook, a stickler for routine and rather irascible. He was proud of his trade, making hand-sewn shoes for West End firms. For many years he had been living in the basement of a friend's house. For about two years preceding admission he had found increasing difficulty in getting on with his work, and had become restless, frequently humming to himself or calling out. His son took him into his own home, and then discovered how very depressed his father was, repeating statements like "I am finished".

The patient was a thin old man, drooling saliva and looking senile without any actual Parkinsonism or memory difficulties. He continually rubbed his hands, and walked up and down the passage of the ward ejaculating, in an apparently stereotyped fashion, expletives like "Blimey", "I am finished" and "Oh Lord". He spoke in a whining voice, but seemed bitter and hostile rather than depressed; sometimes one could not help feeling that he got a perverse satisfaction out of rehearsing the catalogue of his depressive ideas: "I am an impostor", "my pension is gone", "there will be no tomorrow", "you will throw me in the boiler, why not get it over and done with now". He felt something terrible was going to happen; he had not properly opened his bowels or passed water for months. If he let go, there would be "a terrible mess", the consulting room and ultimately the whole hospital would be destroyed by the resulting inundation. At present, faecal matter was only oozing through his pores, and the smell was noticeable to other patients.

After a two months' wait (this was 1949), the patient was given nine ECTs and improved greatly; following relapse he received another seven treatments, and was discharged to his son's home, still bitter and grumbling, but not obviously ill. In spite of much care and suitable occupation, he had to be re-admitted six months later, because an identical clinical picture had gradually developed. On this occasion, general hospital care and occupational therapy was followed by the disappearance of all overt symptoms, but as he was still surly and often restless, he was transferred to a home run by an after-care organisation. After a few months he had to be transferred to a mental hospital because he had run away and had made a suicidal attempt. When visited there, five years later, he was not obviously depressed, and showed only a few isolated failures of memory, though by then he was 81 years old. He worked regularly in the hospital's shoe-repair shop. Though given weekend leaves to visit his son, he had been detained in hospital as his state had remained variable, with many episodes of agitation, hostility and calling-out. He never again expressed bizarre beliefs. He died at the age of 83, following a first cerebral thrombosis.

Long-term follow-up of patients of this type has shown that they do not invariably fail to recover, and that they do not develop senile dementia. In fact, they are merely suffering from a severe and often intractable form of agitated depression.

4. AGITATED DEPRESSIONS

These are by far the commonest affective disorders in middle and late life, and the illnesses may be very severe:

Miss S., aged 66, was admitted soon after retiring from a clerical post, and presented as a grotesquely dishevelled old lady. She continually screwed up her eyes which she believed to be diseased, and she had picked her hands to the extent of producing excoriations. She expressed hopeless ideas, described herself as depressed, but tended to grin rather fatuously. She claimed not to have opened her bowels for months, because they were "all joined up". Food was rotting in her stomach, and she refused to eat any more. "I must be the most unlucky person in the world because I have such dreadful things wrong with me." She frequently tried to retire to bed in order to masturbate. She thought she was not an ordinary person, and that she would never die, but continue her miserable existence for "millions of years".

After five ECTs she made a complete and lasting recovery. Six years later she presented as a frumpish and untidy old woman, tending to smile in a slightly odd, toothy fashion. According to her sister and herself, she was enjoying her retirement, doing a good deal of interesting reading and attending evening classes in history and architecture.

This and many similar patients who make equally good recoveries demonstrate that apparently shallow depressive affect and bizarre delusions do not necessarily foreshadow a chronic course, but again confirm that the clinical concept of senile melancholia is not useful, and that the question of prognosis should be left open by using the non-committal label of severe agitated depression. Almost all patients with anxious-depressive, and therefore agitated, illnesses in late life have a hypochondriacal thought-content. Where the affective disturbance is less severe, hypochondriacal ideas are not usually bizarre and nihilistic, but range from convictions or fears of cancer to unpleasant "fluttering" sensations in the abdomen or chest, which are probably somatic interpretations of anxiety feelings. As anxiety becomes more severe, fears concerning bodily health become increasingly insistent, and in addition patients tend to make reiterative demands for reassurance, to appeal, to importune, and to show agitation. Suicidal risks may be considerable, and especially in suspicious and litigious personalities, paranoid symptoms may be very much in evidence.

The great majority of agitated depressions are mild. No case report is quoted, because they are the bread and butter of clinical psychiatry, frequently seen from middle life onwards and not presenting specifically geriatric features. By contrast, depressions with marked psychomotor retardation are seen rarely in old age, and are almost always exact replicas of illnesses suffered by the patient earlier in his life. Two types of mild agitated depression may be singled out for special study: those following bereavement, and affective disorders arising in patients with long-standing neurotic personality difficulties.

5. REACTIVE DEPRESSIONS

In my experience (Post, 1962), the majority of depressive illnesses in elderly people follow within a few days, weeks or months of some outstanding or incisive occurrence in their lives. In this sense, 67 of 100 consecutively admitted depressives were "reactive", and in 60 patients the precipitating events were actual or threatened losses (acute physical illness: loss of health, in 24; loss of sources of affection: bereavements, serious illness of spouse, removal of children, in 20; and loss of objects: retirement, move from home, loss of property in 16). The presence of the aetiological factor of "loss" in so many elderly depressives is interesting on two accounts. Old age is a period of life when losses of the kind suffered by our patients are the order of the day, and this may well be one of the reasons why the occurrence of first depressions is so often postponed into late life. Related to the frequency of external causal events, a positive family history of the affective reaction type was less often obtained in late onset depression than in patients with first attacks occurring before the age of 50 (family history in patients with first attack before 50, positive in 80 per cent; onset 50–65, 63 per cent; onset after 65, 44 per cent). Other workers report similar findings (Kay, 1959; Stenstedt, 1959), and there exists a body of opinion according to which external causes are more important, and heredo-genetic factors less powerful in depressions of late life than in those seen in younger patients. Returning to the precipitating role of "loss", we should recall that according to psychoanalytic theory, many depressive illnesses are caused by the loss of external sources of self-esteem in certain people (with pregenital fixations and narcissistic orientations). Impairment of physical health, loss or threatened loss of loving relations, impairment of status on retiring, and loss of home or property, which had occurred in some 60 per cent of my sample of elderly depressives, represent precisely such losses of sources of self-esteem. I may add that only some 15 per cent of my group of depressives were entirely free of neurotic personality traits, and that many had shown obsessive-phobic trends, which are said to be linked to pregenital libidinal fixation. Furthermore, in 40 per cent of patients there had been definite sexual maladjustment in earlier life. So all the ingredients of the Freudian recipe for depression were frequently present in this sample of patients.

Starting from psychoanalytic premises, a group of workers (their work was summarised by Stern, 1954) studied elderly patients with grief reactions. They thought that in many instances old people developed physical symptoms rather than overt depressions, and that, instead of being self-accusatory, they tended to displace their hostile feelings about the lost person (who was often idealised) towards their surviving friends. This reaction was explained by suggesting that the ego is weakened by age, and that feelings of depression and guilt produced by a further cutting off of sources of self-esteem might not be tolerated. However, overt depressions following bereavement are suffered by many elderly people, and the classical Freudian mechanisms linking melancholia with mourning are sometimes fairly clearly discerned, as in a recent (slightly disguised) case:

> Mrs. W., aged 66, had lost her husband five months earlier after nursing him through his last illness, cancer of the stomach. A few days after his death she had taken an overdose of sleeping tablets, but was soon discharged from a general hospital. Her family doctor finally referred the patient to my out-patient clinic, because she had been unable to hold down a job and had complained of difficulties with swallowing. The patient was only mildly depressed, but in view of the past suicidal attempt, and the fact that she was living alone and in lonely circumstances, I thought it wiser to admit her.

On closer inquiry, the following story emerged: the patient and her husband had only married when she was 36 years old, and after a courtship lasting eight years. Marriage had been delayed for allegedly economic reasons, and only occurred after the husband had had a nervous breakdown. There were no children, though sexual relations were said to have been "all right". Husband and wife worked together in their shop, and had very few social contacts. Relatives on both sides attended the husband's funeral, but following this the patient's contacts with members of her family had been brief, rare and superficial. This patient felt that her inability to concentrate at work and her depression were due to a decision on her part to be emotionally dead, after her friends had discouraged her talking to them about her husband and her own sad state. It was suspected that this attitude, as well as her suicidal attempt, were attempts at identifying with her dead husband, and that these mechanisms had been resorted to by the patient because she had not been allowed to carry on the work of mourning, which consists of cutting the links with a lost person. The patient was accordingly encouraged to ventilate her thoughts and feelings. Identification with the dead husband was confirmed when in discussing her fears of not being able to swallow the patient disclosed, not perhaps surprisingly, that her husband had had difficulties in swallowing in his last illness. She began to blame herself for various things she had done or left undone while nursing him. She felt guilty about getting her husband to sign documents in connection with the sale of their business, when he was no longer capable of understanding what he was doing. Psychoanalytic theory suggests that self-reproaches of this sort are really hostile feelings against the dead (introjected) lost person, and it gradually became clear that the patient's feelings towards her husband had been strongly ambivalent. The couple's prolonged courtship had been due to her disliking many aspects of a more intimate relationship with him, and she resented being emotionally blackmailed into a marriage, which was not as ideal as had been claimed originally. No explicit interpretations were offered to this patient, but she cried a good deal during the interviews. Whether this treatment or the further passage of time led to her improvement and ultimate recovery, is impossible to say. In most cases, Freudian mechanisms are less clearly seen, and there certainly are many patients with depressions following bereavement, who are not helped by ventilating their ambivalent feelings. Quite often their illnesses, though reactive and psychodynamically understandable, are of psychotic intensity and type, with difficulties in communication precluding psychotherapeutic exploration and management in hospital practice.

6. NEUROTIC DEPRESSIONS

These are disorders for which there are almost as many definitions as there are psychiatrists! The term is often used as synonymous with reactive depression, especially for those illnesses in which psychogenic factors are clearly discerned, and reflected in the symptomatology. Other writers call "neurotic" all depressive illnesses which are mild and "non-psychotic", i.e. not associated with marked loss of weight, early morning waking, guilt feelings and a mental content of delusional quality. I suggest we use the term simply to denote depressive illnesses occurring in people with long-standing and fairly well-defined phobic, obsessive or hysterical propensities. This background neurosis has not necessarily been sufficiently incapacitating to urge the patient towards any form of treatment, but in the wake of depressive disturbances the neurotic symptoms often become more severe. Occasionally they even change into delusions, as in the case of an obsessional man who had had a lifelong fear that past masturbation might eventually cause a disease of his spine. He was an educated man, familiar with sensible writings on this subject, and he realised that his fear was unfounded, and—as he quite rightly said—an obsession. And yet, during at least one of his depressions, he for a time was firmly and unshakeably convinced that his spine was "decaying". As a general rule, however, the depressive illnesses of neurotic persons tend to be mild, and to lack psychotic-delusional features in their symptomatology.

Depressive illnesses in a setting of lifelong neurosis, the neurotic symptoms continuing in a more or less unchanged fashion after each affective episode, were seen in 21 per cent of elderly depressives requiring admission. Neurotic depressions are even more commonly encountered in out-patient and general practice. Much more rarely, manic attacks may occur as well. A case record may serve to illustrate the relationship between depressive illnesses and a neurotic life history. It is an example of the commonest combination, viz. between affective illnesses and obsessional neurosis. Much evidence suggests that there are linkages between the affective reaction type and obsessional neurosis, both on heredogenetic and on psychodynamic grounds. The depressions of obsessionals are often severe and acute, and sometimes respond quickly to electroconvulsive therapy.

Mr. H. was a retired naval officer. One of his sisters had "compulsive cleaning régimes", a brother had had several depressive breakdowns, and both his children had as adults had psychoanalytic treatment for affective disorders and personality problems. In childhood he had marked fears of the dark and of thunderstorms, and later on this well-connected and intelligent man pursued an only moderately successful career in the navy, probably because he was noted for being indecisive, pessimistic, over-cautious and given to self-blame. He had no real friends outside his family, and was over-dependent on his wife, who was loyal but had remained sexually unsatisfied by the patient.

At the age of 45 obsessional closing of doors was first noted.

At 59, one month after retirement, he became sleepless, lost weight, was despondent, restless and preoccupied with imaginary financial difficulties (he had ample independent means). The checking of bolts and locks on doors became a much greater problem, and he also became obsessionally preoccupied with light switches and fires. He recovered gradually after one year, but was never again entirely free of these obsessional symptoms.

When aged 64 he had an identical illness; he was treated in a neurosis hospital by psychotherapy, and improved after six months.

At 69, 71 and 74, he had similar attacks, each responding promptly to ECT given as an out-patient after illnesses lasting only three months.

At the age of 75, out-patient ECT appeared to fail, and the patient was for the first time admitted under my care. He was not obviously retarded or agitated in behaviour or talk, but exhibited a facial tic. Though not suicidal, he was moderately depressed, as well as mildly self-depreciatory, and concerned over his financial situation. He exhibited a tapping compulsion in addition to the habits already described, which he called foolish. He finally improved after a few more ECTs, but this illness had lasted 9 months. It was necessary to support him as an out-patient, and at 76 he had to be re-admitted for 9 months; it was not at all clear whether ECT was responsible for his eventual recovery. He remained surprisingly well for some three years. He gained weight and slept without drugs for long periods, with his obsessional symptoms being hardly a problem.

At 80, all his symptoms returned, and in spite of two sets of ECT recovery did not occur for 14 months.

At 82 he had to be re-admitted, and responded promptly to ECT after only 5 months of actual illness.

At 85 this experience was exactly repeated. He died 18 months later without developing further depressive symptoms.

Almost all attacks appeared to have been triggered off by external events, such as excessive demands made by a Civil Defence job, by domestic problems, or recurrent attacks of bronchopneumonia. From the age of 80 the patient showed rapidly increasing physical senility, but in life as well as in his performance of psychological tests there was no significant falling off in mental abilities, and, except immediately after the numerous convulsive therapies, there was no memory impairment.

7. "MASKED" DEPRESSIONS

In the case of so-called neurotic depressions, affective symptoms always stand out very clearly against the background of neurosis. By contrast, there are probably many elderly people with long-standing neurotic complaints, where underlying depressions fail to be recognised. No illustrative case records will be presented because it is never possible to produce convincing evidence for the existence of these depressive elements. One's experience that some neurotic conditions in middle and late life improve greatly during the administration of anti-depressive drugs does not necessarily prove *ex post facto* that an affective disorder had been present. Personally, I always think it worth while to give these preparations a thorough trial in complaint disorders, especially long-standing hypochondriasis, when in the course of a long neurotic story there appear to be some new developments, such as slight changes of sleep pattern (e.g. need for increased night sedation), weight, interests and activities. Other psychiatrists may object, very justifiably, that the concept of affective illness would be stretched too far if it were made to cover variations in severity of chronic personality disorders.

However, many undoubted depressions of mild or moderate severity remain unrecognised during part or the whole of their course. Families and family doctors may be notoriously slow to realise that an elderly person is pathologically depressed. In two different samples of affective patients over 60, only one-fifth had been referred to psychiatrists relatively early, i.e. during the first six months of illness. In most patients, it took from 6 to 18 months before the need for specialist treatment was felt. As it seems unlikely that general practitioners would continue to treat without success depressives for more than a few weeks before referring them to consultants (certainly, in the years before the recent flood of tranquillising and so-called anti-depressive drugs), it is difficult to avoid the conclusion that the presence or gravity of these illnesses had gone unrecognised by doctors and families for many months. I shall refrain from quoting cases, as it is always easy to be wise after the event.

In a representative random sample of old people comprising 271 persons over 65 living in the community, Parsons (1962) found two people suffering at the time of the survey from depressive illnesses which had not been recognised by their relatives or medical attendants. In fact, the daughter of one took a rather unsympathetic attitude; he had nothing to be depressed about, and therefore he could not possibly be depressed. This patient seemed on the way towards recovery. The other case may be quoted (with the investigator's kind permission):

> He was a bachelor of 67 living with his in-laws. In 1919 he was discharged from the army, allegedly on account of malaria. However, he had at no time been given a pension, and admitted that at the time he had also been "nervy". For a while he was observed to go about with a scarf over his nose, so that people should not see it, but by 1922 this behaviour had ceased. Many years later he attended his GP to have a cut in his wrist stitched, claiming that a car had hit him! Some four years before the date of the survey, this man began to complain of an unpleasant taste in his mouth, and was sent to a consultant physician who declared himself unable to explain this symptom. Three years later, his symptoms were still continuing, and he was sent to an ear-nose-and-throat surgeon, to whom he complained of fullness in his left nostril and a nasty taste in his mouth. Full clinical and X-ray investigations were negative; the symptoms were regarded as functional, and reassurance was advised.
> When he was interviewed, the following record of the man's complaints was obtained: "Nasty taste coming from the back of my throat the last eight months. It's on my mind all the time. It's like an obstruction going from my mouth to my left ear. I dwell on the fact that I can't do what I used to do." He also had a full feeling in his head, and felt worst in the mornings, having slept poorly with early waking for some time. He was depressed: "There is no way out of it. If I won a lot of money, it wouldn't buck me up." He was self-belittling and seemed puzzled and agitated.

A patient seen on the very day on which the present section was drafted, reminds me to point out that family doctors often fail to recognise depressive illnesses, even when there have been recent similar attacks. The patient in question had had a first illness at the age of 68, which had been characterised by loss of appetite, trembling sensations in his stomach, loss of interest, lack of concentration with depression and sleeping difficulties developing gradually. After the usual period in a general hospital for fruitless gastric investigations, the patient finally came under psychiatric care some 18 months after the onset of ill health. Full recovery occurred after two sets of ECT and four months in hospital. It was maintained for more than four years, when the patient was brought along by his wife bearing the following letter from the family doctor: "This man came to see me last Thursday complaining of severe stomach pains for which I could find no obvious cause. His wife I understand has now taken the matter out of my hands and made an appointment for him to see you tomorrow. . . ." The patient's wife reported that he had been perfectly well until suffering from a painful ear infection which was successfully treated by his doctor, but that he had then become sleepless and restless, and had lost all interest in television.

I: "But I thought he had to see his doctor on account of severe stomach pains?"

Wife: "Stomach pains? Them were no real stomach pains! Just his stomach turning over all the time, just as he had four years ago."

She decided her husband was psychiatrically ill again and took the undiplomatic action described in the doctor's letter. The patient presented an identical picture to that in his previous illness (he again recovered fully following electroconvulsive therapy).

Both these patients presented with physical complaints. The great frequency of hypochondriacal symptoms in the depressions of the elderly was confirmed in a study of 152 consecutive depressives admitted under my care (de Alarcón, in preparation). Hypochondriasis, either in the form of unjustified physical complaints or of a conviction of suffering from a physical illness, was found in 65 per cent of men and in 62 per cent of women. In some the depression had been truly masked in that the illness had started with bodily complaints, and several weeks or months had passed in one-quarter of cases before symptoms more clearly indicative of a depressive mood had appeared. In the majority, hypochondriasis had dominated the picture, but depression had been present all the time, though noticeable only to a psychiatrically-aware doctor. Contrary to expectation, only 20 per cent of these hypochondriacal depressives had shown unusual concerns over their physical health before they fell ill. Therefore, the occurrence of hypochondriacal symptoms in elderly people, for the first time in life, should be a warning signal to look out for evidence of depression, after physical examination has failed to reveal disease or to point to a clear need for further investigations. It is especially imperative to recognise depression underlying hypochondriacal complaints, because suicidal tendencies were far commoner in hypochondriacal depressives (1 in every 4) than in other affectively ill patients (1 in 15).

Affective disorder may be an important but unrecognised factor in chronic physical illness, and attention was recently drawn to this by geriatric physicians (Wilson and Lawson, 1962). These workers noticed that there was among their admissions a group of people who were miserable, gloomy, taken up with themselves and with their bodily complaints. There was no suicidal intent, but they blamed the environment for feelings that they would like to be dead. There was no guilt or self-reproach: on the contrary, they thought that things had gone against them, but that they themselves had done their best. Almost all these patients were widowed, but in comfortable circumstances and regularly visited. In spite of this, feelings of loneliness were common, and these were often associated with actual and confirmed hostility felt by other members of their families. It seemed to the authors that rejection by the children was associated with faulty attitudes on the part of the old people themselves, which included desires to dominate, unreasonable demands for attention, or frank hostility. In three-quarters of cases there was evidence of lifelong personality difficulties or neurotic trends which had, however, not grossly affected their earlier lives; it was noted that their reactions to bereavement had been prolonged. Most of these patients had been more or less bedridden for several months or even years, but their depressions responded surprisingly and unexpectedly within a few days of admission to hospital, long before their physical disorders had been effectively dealt with. In fact, relief of depression was thought to be due to relief of physical symptoms in only one-third of cases. Non-specific aspects of care in an active medical unit, and the firm rejection of self-pity, as well as the restoration of self-respect involved in getting the patient up and properly dressed, were regarded as the effective therapeutic agents. These people all had significant physical illnesses: 10 of 23 patients died during the subsequent two years. A few developed minor senile mental changes, and one-third relapsed into depressive states, but none attempted or committed suicide.

This section on "masked" depressions and invalid reactions has brought our discussion round full circle to mild mood disorders of old people, which are hardly ever seen by psychiatrists, and about whose natural history we know next to nothing. We will conclude this chapter by discussing the outlook in the more clearly defined affective illnesses. Their natural history remains unknown, as sooner or later their course is influenced by treatment.

THE OUTLOOK IN AFFECTIVE ILLNESSES

1. MANIA

In manic disorders the outlook is well known and varies little. Patients tend to remain disturbed somewhat longer than is the case at an earlier age, but most attacks subside within a few weeks, and they rarely last much longer than six months. Every mental hospital sports one or two cases of chronic mania. Their illnesses have not as a rule started in old age, but during the fifth or sixth decade of life. Modern treatment with phenothiazine drugs, which control the severity of the symptoms but probably not their duration, does not appear to affect the tendency of manic disorders to recur almost invariably. In the elderly attacks tend to be frequent, most commonly every 1–2 years. Especially when the first attack has shown marked depressive admixtures, some subsequent illnesses will almost certainly be either mixed or clearly melancholic. Later illnesses are not necessarily more severe or prolonged than first ones, and the intervals between them do not always become shorter. Beyond the certainty of recurrence, nothing can be predicted about the future of patients exhibiting manic symptoms, because these conditions are relatively uncommon, and it has not been possible to follow up patients in sufficiently large numbers.

2. DEPRESSION

Much more is known about the future lives of patients suffering from depressive illnesses after the age of 60. Not so long ago, senile depressions were thought to carry a very poor prognosis. They were looked upon as chronic disorders during which patients were prone to succumb to intercurrent physical illnesses, and it was held that senile melancholia was frequently the first stage of senile or arteriosclerotic dementia. Recoveries were known to occur, but it was feared that they were only rarely complete, that recurrences were almost the rule, and likely to be followed by increasing emotional enfeeblement.

The care of these agitated patients with their food refusals, their reiterative and importuning demands, and their aggravating hypochondriacal talk, used to impose a severe strain on relatives, doctors and nurses. Following its introduction some twenty-five years ago, electroconvulsive therapy was at first only reluctantly employed in elderly depressives, until it became established that this form of treatment was but rarely contra-indicated by physical disabilities, and never by age alone. From being a tedious and disheartening task, the "active" treatment of senile depression with convulsive, occupational and social therapies was found to achieve very encouraging results. Moreover, pre-frontal leucotomy was often successful in patients where these treatments had failed. Length of hospital stay was shortened considerably. In a large regional mental hospital only 32 per cent of depressive patients over 60 became fit for discharge in the first six months following admission during the years 1934–6; in the years 1948–9, this proportion had risen to just under 60 per cent (Roth, 1955). In my own unit at a teaching hospital, where patients tend to come from more favourable social backgrounds, 88 per cent of elderly depressives became fit for discharge some ten years ago.

However, I checked on these encouraging immediate results by personally following my patients over the subsequent six years (Post, 1962). It then emerged that during this period (which in one-third of subjects had been shortened by death) only 28 per cent had remained free of further affective symptoms. The majority of patients suffered further affective breakdowns, from which they did not always recover, and in some a personality change was noted in the direction of greater moodiness, increasing social withdrawal and hypochondriacal invalidism. Also, it turned out that 14 per cent of patients never recovered at all, but remained psychotic during practically the whole of the follow-up period. An attempt was made to evaluate the outcome of affective illness in this sample of relatively favourably placed elderly people by taking account not only of the persistence or recurrence of symptoms, but also of the amount of illness and the level of social adjustment during subsequent life. Really satisfactory results had been achieved in only 19 per cent of patients, in that they had been psychiatrically ill for only short periods, had made complete recoveries, and had maintained or even improved their general adjustment. Thirty-five per cent had been ill for longer periods, had not always recovered completely, but had maintained their earlier level of social adjustment. Twenty-eight per cent never recovered fully, but deteriorated only slightly in the social sphere, almost always because they were supported by their families; but 18 per cent suffered from mental symptoms almost continuously, and had in addition become increasingly isolated and ill-adjusted in their environment. Investigation of a later sample of elderly patients (Colwell and Post, 1959) confirmed that the long-term outlook in senile depression was far less favourable than superficial impressions suggest; during the first two years following treatment, only 21 per cent of patients remained free of symptoms, and 70 per cent received further medical attention for affective symptoms. As was pointed out earlier, one very reassuring fact has clearly emerged from a number of recent (including our own) investigations; contrary to expectation, elderly depressives develop senile or arteriosclerotic brain deterioration no more frequently than other old people.

The present position may thus be summarised as follows:

(1) The affective illnesses of old age are unrelated to the senile and arteriosclerotic dementias; affective symptoms are only rarely the prodromata of as yet hidden pathological processes in the brain.

(2) Modern methods of treatment achieve relief of symptoms in the great majority of elderly depressives.

(3) Unfortunately, immediate relief is followed by varying degrees of psychological and social invalidism in about one-half of cases. The impact which tranquillising and anti-depressive drugs may have made on chronic or frequently recurring depressive illnesses has not so far been satisfactorily determined.

In the preceding section of this chapter we described a variety of depressive clinical pictures. Classification was employed to facilitate this description, but as we went along it became increasingly clear that no essential differences existed between the various types apart from degree of severity. We now have to add that very few predictions of the likely response to treatment can be made from the type of clinical picture with one single exception: patients with brain damage, i.e. with definite neurological signs and symptoms, and/or definite dementia when first seen, only rarely make full and lasting recoveries from depressive breakdowns. Apart from the occurrence of further cerebral deterioration, they either do not lose their affective symptoms at all, or show a depressive personality change and invalidism, usually associated with frequent recurrence of more disabling depressive symptoms. Perhaps the outlook is a little better in patients with severe and clear-cut melancholic symptoms (guilt delusions and convincingly communicated depressive affect), especially when they have suffered similar melancholic illnesses earlier in life independently of any cerebral deterioration.

We may attempt to differentiate in terms of aetiology, symptomatology, course and prognosis between manic-depressive depressions, involutional depressions and senile melancholias. However, we noted earlier that depressive illnesses occurring for the first time late in the senium ("senile melancholias") did not differ as far as their symptoms were concerned from conditions occurring earlier, and that they did not become necessarily chronic or ended in dementia. In fact, bizarre hypochondriacal, nihilistic delusions and ideas of enormity, especially in the area of guilt, may occur at earlier ages, and in common with all symptoms indicating severe and acute mental aberration, are if anything of favourable prognostic portent. The concept of "involutional melancholia" has had a checkered career in psychiatry during the last seventy years; it was abandoned by its originator, Kraepelin, but was later reformulated on several occasions. The term customarily refers to agitated depressions occurring for the first time in life after the age 45–50, in contrast to manic-depressive illnesses which manifest themselves at an earlier age. Involutional depressions are also said to pursue a much more prolonged course, and it is often suggested that when remissions are produced by treatment, recurrences are frequent or that there ensues a state of mental invalidism, with hypochondriasis and social withdrawal as its main features. In involutional depression, a typical pre-morbid personality has been alleged, characterised by obsessionality, rigidity of outlook, inhibition or maladjustment in the sexual sphere, parsimoniousness, temperamental coldness and introversion. One can always point out a few patients who are fully representative of the stereotype of involutional melancholia, but from a genetic point of view (Stenstedt, 1959) and seen in context with elderly depressives as a group (Post, 1962) the typical picture is but rarely encountered. Agitated hypochondriacal depression is, in fact, the commonest affective disorder, in this country and during the present century, in persons over the age of 50. However, age of onset, symptomatology and response to treatment are, as we have seen, anything but uniform. Elderly depressives are frequently said to have had obsessional and rigid personalities earlier in life, but traits of this kind are also associated with other disorders requiring mental hospital admission in old age, e.g. senile dementia. The position of "paranoid involutional psychosis" will be discussed in the next chapter, concerned with the significance of schizophrenic symptoms. The presence of paranoid symptoms is not, as a rule, an ominous feature in elderly depressives.

One is led to conclude regretfully that it is not possible to differentiate depressive patients with good outcome from those with a poorer prognosis on the basis of their belonging to separate disease entities like manic-depressive, involutional or senile depressions. On the other hand, a number of prognostic factors have emerged which may prove to have limited clinical usefulness. The following features tend to be favourable: age, at time of illness, below 70; a positive family history for affective disorders; recovery from earlier attacks before the age of 50, especially where they had been sufficiently severe to require admissions to hospital; an extroverted personality with social ties and activities reaching beyond the family; an even temperament, without cyclothymic or dysthymic trends; and in the clinical picture, severe, and even schizophreniform, symptoms. Unfavourable features are pathological brain changes, and, indeed, any serious and disabling disease in any part of the body; also a general appearance of senile decrepitude, especially in women over 70. All these features differentiated patients with good outcome from those with poor responses to treatment more often than might be expected by chance, but there were, of course, many patients who were exceptions, and the features just enumerated are thus of little help in the prognosis of individual cases. There are, however, two features which were found to have been much more useful indicators of outcome: patients hardly ever did well if they had been uninterruptedly ill with depression for more than two years; by contrast, complete remission of all symptoms at completion of treatment was almost always followed by long periods of good mental health, but many women, provided they were under 70, also did well, even though at the time of discharge they still had some residual symptoms (Post, 1962).

In conclusion, it should be stressed that considerations of long-term prognosis should not influence us unduly. Affective illnesses are very unpleasant, and much distress can be avoided by their prompt recognition and treatment, even if the results are not always entirely satisfactory or lasting, and if on account of a long history or the presence of cerebral or other disease only partial improvement may be obtained in most cases. The presence of affective symptoms is usually recognised easily once their possibility is constantly kept in mind and specific inquiries are made.

CHAPTER V

PARANOID SYNDROMES

NOSOLOGICAL DIFFICULTIES

Literally translated, paranoia means derangement of mind, and paranoid, crazy. In clinical usage this term has become almost synonymous with persecutory, but it may more generally refer to all kinds of experiences in which a person falsely or to an exaggerated extent believes himself the object of attention from others. This feeling may amount to a habitual attitude, by which belittlement and hostility by other people are taken for granted, and which may be maintained with considerable conviction by sensitive or paranoid personalities. Episodic impressions of undue attention from others, which are evaluated as improbable or puzzling, are termed ideas of reference. More persistent experiences of self-reference, the reality of which is doubted but of which a person cannot rid himself, are sometimes called over-valued ideas; they are not necessarily paranoid, but may be hypochondriacal in content. Finally, paranoid beliefs may be held with unshakable conviction, when it is customary to speak of paranoid delusions.

The content and form of paranoid experiencing depend on the setting in which they occur. Sensitive personalities tend to view other persons from a position of inferiority, whereas litigious persons assume a position of strength, from which they fight back against their imagined adversaries. Outside the area of their preoccupations, the behaviour of paranoid personalities is not necessarily disordered, and their attitudes are at least remotely related to some reality situation. Some social settings are alleged to be especially conducive to paranoid experiencing and behaviour: the immigrant status, the atmosphere of a police state, economically dependent spinsterhood, partial deafness—to mention only a few. Paranoid interpretations may also occur when reality testing is impaired, in states of altered awareness, due to severe emotional disturbances, acute organic confusional states or dementing processes. Ideas of reference and over-valued ideas are encountered in relatively mild or incipient psychiatric illnesses. With predominantly anxious or depressive affects, they are of depreciatory content; self-enhancing and wishful ideas (e.g. the impression of being loved or desired) are experienced in a setting of elated or euphoric moods. Paranoid delusions in a setting of depression may be held as directed against a self which is felt to be wicked, guilty, worthless and deserving of punishment. Or, their content may indicate that the patient believes himself to be in a position of superiority, envied by others; in this case, his mood is likely to be an elated one (manic), an euphoric one (organic or schizophrenic), or an ecstatic one (schizophrenic). In many schizophrenic illnesses, paranoid experiences lack any obvious affective colouring. Here, they may take the form (more frequently than in other psychoses) of true auditory hallucinations, often a running commentary on his activities. Paranoid experiences in schizophrenics may occur as signs, messages, thought-intrusions, feelings of influence and passivity—some of the phenomena interpreted as indicating splitting of the personality and dissolution of ego boundaries.

Paranoid symptoms in the elderly may differ widely in diagnostic significance. They may be part of a senile character change, and they may be caused by acute and chronic brain syndromes. Depressive and manic illnesses in the aged are sometimes associated with severe persecutory or grandiose delusions, which disappear on recovery from the affective disorder. Finally, there are paranoid illnesses which run a chronic course (if untreated), and which are not associated with undue intellectual impairment. A great variety of names has been given to this last group of disorders, indicating the considerable uncertainty of their nosological position: senile paranoid reaction or paranoid state; senile paranoia, "involutionsparanoia"; senile paraphrenia or late paraphrenia; paranoid schizophrenia, symptomatic schizophrenia, or senile schizophreniform psychosis.

A brief discussion of this controversial, and at present largely academic, matter will not lead us too far from our subject. Personally, I would like to restrict the terms paranoid state or paranoid reaction to conditions which are transitory, but at the same time not associated with organic confusional or affective disorders. As far as their occurrence in elderly patients is concerned, I am not aware of any long-term studies confirming their temporary, and possibly reactive, nature. Paranoia was a term originally reserved for delusional illnesses, which were persistent and well systematised; but the claim that patients with these conditions failed to develop schizophrenic symptoms outside their delusional system of ideas was not confirmed by follow-up studies. Paranoia was, therefore, incorporated with paraphrenia, an illness characterised not only by paranoid delusions, but also (not invariably, though) by auditory hallucinations. Paraphrenia was thought to differ from paranoid schizophrenia on account of the absence of schizophrenic deterioration of affect and volition; the personality was thought to remain intact. Later on, it was shown that there were no differences between paraphrenics and paranoid schizophrenics in the structure of symptoms, course of disorder, or hereditary mechanisms. Continued freedom from affective incongruity or flattening, from catatonic features, stereotypies, and other volitional disorders was attributed to the higher age of onset in the paraphrenic type of paranoid schizophrenic. Similar considerations demolished in the eyes of many the concept of "involutionsparanoia". Readers interested in these developments of psychiatric thought are referred to Kolle's (1931) monograph and to Mayer-Gross's (1932) clarifying chapter in Bumke's *Handbuch*. It seems unlikely, however, that the riddle of schizophrenia will be solved by juggling with observations of symptoms, clinical records, or family histories based on other people's diagnoses. For this reason, I do not wish to review the controversy as to whether there are valid distinctions between patients with nuclear or process schizophrenic symptoms and those with schizophreniform symptoms only (Langfeldt, 1960). The terms "schizophrenia-like psychosis" and "symptomatic schizophrenia" have been applied to patients who are held to suffer from a basic non-schizophrenic illness, such as epilepsy, GPI, cerebral tumour, amphetamine intoxication, etc. This terminology is, therefore, of special relevance to the paranoid psychoses of old age, in which underlying brain changes are often suspected. Slater, Beard & Clithero (1963) have defended the concept of schizophrenia-like psychosis associated with chronic epilepsy mainly on genetic-hereditary grounds; 69 patients mustered between them only 2 schizophrenics among first degree relatives, whereas the familes of 69 true schizophrenics would have contained an expected number of about 17 secondary cases. In addition, there was no excess of schizoid previous personalities in their epileptics with schizophrenia-like psychoses, 75 per cent of whom had a special kind of epilepsy (temporal lobe). In the great majority of their cases, symptomatology and course were of the paraphrenic type, with good preservation of affect and other personality functions. (This finding may perhaps be explained by the relatively late onset of mental symptoms, at an average age of 30 years). Slater's work, as well as that of other recent investigators, showed clearly that no distinction between schizophrenia-like psychoses, symptomatic schizophrenias, or process schizophrenias could be made on the basis of the psychiatric picture. Process symptoms of a paranoid type, i.e. passivity feelings, influence experiences, and depersonalisation, were frequently encountered in so-called symptomatic schizophrenias.

Until we have gained a better understanding of the true causes of the paranoid-schizophrenic reaction-type, any elaborate classification appears to be an unscientific and pretentious practice. This view applies with special force to the schizophrenias of old age, whose study has only recently begun. Bleuler (1943), in his review, reported that a mere 15 per cent of schizophrenias started after the age of 40, and only 5 per cent after 60. Only 4 of Mueller's (1959) 101 schizophrenics (followed into their senium) became ill after the age of 60. Among elderly psychiatric patients admitted to the Heidelberg Clinic, Lechler (1950) found that 8 per cent suffered from schizophreniform paranoid symptoms. Janzarik (1957) and Hirschmann and Klages (1957) had each been able to study 50 late schizophrenics. Fish (1960) reported that 41 of 264 consecutive senile psychiatric admissions in Edinburgh were suffering from paranoid illnesses, but he diagnosed as schizophrenic only 16 (of whom 7 fell ill after the age of 60). Most earlier investigators had not examined their patients at the time of admission, or had only followed them personally over short periods. However, Kay and Roth (1961) were able to study 99 patients with what they call "late paraphrenia", none of whom had fallen ill before the age of 55. Forty-two were personally examined on admission, and all 99 cases were followed up over long periods.

We shall return to the findings of these investigations. They have been enumerated at this stage to demonstrate the recency of work in this field. For this reason, and on account of the unsatisfactory state of our knowledge, I propose not to use any elaborate classification of the schizophrenias of old age in this book. On the contrary, a naïve position will be purposely adopted, in that a series of clinical pictures will be described, graded simply according to the amount of personality involvement by paranoid or schizophrenic experiences and behaviour, as well as in relation to the presence of brain changes and of sensory defects.

CLINICAL FEATURES

(1) *Paranoid personality developments.* Elderly people who have become increasingly suspicious and cantankerous hardly ever reach psychiatrists. They are known to us largely through the complaints of their friends, but one suspects that they make up a large proportion of the eccentric personalities described by family doctors and general physicians in various surveys of old people living in their own homes. They are usually spinsters and bachelors, or people whose marriages broke up early in life. They have gradually withdrawn from society, often after quarrelling with their few remaining relatives. They are rarely seen by anybody, and several days may pass before serious illness or death are noticed by their neighbours. Psychiatrists are more familiar with

(2) *Acute paranoid reactions* to social stresses which may affect people with sensitive and dependent personalities. They are perhaps related to Kretschmer's sensitive reactions.

> Mr. E., aged 72, came from a healthy family, and had himself never suffered from nervous symptoms. Though placid, he had always been shy and reserved. He married in his late thirties a wife who was a few years older, and a rheumatic semi-invalid. Following retirement, he had devoted himself solely to the care of his wife, who died one year before his admission became necessary. He felt lonely, but looked after himself adequately, paying regular visits to a sister. However, after a few months he began to complain that teddy boys were getting into his flat. He avoided being out after dark, because he felt that people were in the street talking about him and saying that they were going to cut off his head. Neighbours and police investigated his complaints with negative results on several occasions. Finally he was convinced that an assault was imminent, and he decided to take his life rather than fall into the hands of his persecutors. He made a poor attempt at cutting his throat, thought the better of it, and presented himself at a hospital department. On admission he was not depressed, but frightened and convinced of the reality of his experiences. He slept well and developed no paranoid symptoms in hospital. After being placed on increasing doses of a

phenothiazine drug, he went home for weekends, and reported absence of any disturbances. The psychiatric social worker helped him to find a part-time job, and mobilised other people in the house into giving the patient friendly support. However, following discharge after 3½ months in hospital, he failed to avail himself of these arrangements, did not take his tablets, felt he could not stay in his flat and clamoured for re-admission. He refused to go into a home for elderly people, and tried once again to live in his flat. In spite of taking his tablets and continued social support, recurrence of florid paranoid symptoms necessitated his re-admission. His symptoms subsided at once, and he was settled in a Home, where after initial grumbles he became quite happy and satisfied. He remained free of all symptoms without any drug treatment up to the time of writing, i.e. 2½ years later. He never accepted that his experiences had been imaginary, but showed no intellectual or personality changes.

In the case of this and many similar patients, there arises a strong impression that psychogenic mechanisms, akin to hysterical reactions to stress, are at work. The symptoms are not bizarre, but in the context in which they occur quite understandable, if somewhat sensational. They cease as soon as stress is relieved, and they fail to occur as soon as patients are placed in socially sheltered positions. Personalities affected in this way tend to be dependent and sensitive, but quite frequently persecutory symptoms arise in old people of combative spirit, and they cannot then be regarded as escape from stress.

Mrs. E. had always been an outgoing person with many superficial friends. Up to the age of 72, she had been working in several London theatres as a dresser. She had been married and widowed twice, but was only in intermittent contact with her two sons, as she did not get on with her daughters-in-law. Soon after retirement from a career which was allegedly enriched by many phantastic and probably phantasied back-stage episodes, she began to complain that the people upstairs made noises to annoy her; apparently she got quite disturbed following an angry scene. She settled down for a while at a different address, but then began to complain that her coal was stolen, and that children broke into her room and damaged her belongings. This was done at the instigation of neighbours who envied her higher social status. Frequent visits to the local police station finally resulted in her compulsory admission to a mental observation ward. Neither there, nor following transfer to our treatment unit, did she show any abnormal behaviour or fresh paranoid symptoms; nor was she anxious, depressed, or sleepless. She had never experienced any hallucinations, passivity feelings, or other schizophrenic phenomena. She was discharged after two months, and found herself new accommodation. Soon she failed to keep appointments for supportive interviews. Three years later, her son reported: ". . . my mother's condition continues to fluctuate, one moment she will be 100 per cent, next she gets the idea that some person or persons are stealing or damaging her belongings. Since leaving the Bethlem she has made nine or ten moves into furnished rooms . . ."

(3) *Paranoid illnesses associated with sensory and cerebral defects.*
Deafness has been shown to be significantly more common in
paranoid than in non-paranoid mental patients (Houston & Royse,
1954), and it has been suggested that impairment of verbal communications on account of deafness or of linguistic difficulties renders
susceptible persons more suspicious, and more prone to persecutory
interpretations. Incapacitating deafness was more common in elderly
paranoid patients (25 per cent) than in elderly depressives (11 per
cent) (Post, 1962a). However, only 75 per cent of deaf paranoid
seniles suffered from auditory hallucinations (as against 60 per cent
of the non-deaf). While hearing disorders and tinnitus may increase a
tendency towards paranoid symptoms and auditory hallucinations,
the importance of this relationship should not be overstressed. Most
deaf old people do not come to feel persecuted. Many, however, may
complain of hearing noises or even voices. Sometimes they may begin
to believe in their reality:

> Miss W., aged 76, was described as a confirmed spinster, of strict morals and
> meticulous tidiness. Up to the age of 67 she had worked regularly in domestic
> service, and she had never suffered any physical or emotional illnesses.
> Following retirement she had gone to live in a single furnished room, but
> visited one of her nieces quite frequently. From the age of 72, she had
> gradually become increasingly deaf as well as inconvenienced by tinnitus. She
> used a hearing aid well, but a few months before admission she had begun to
> hear light music, which she realised was imaginary and which she regarded as
> a rather amusing phenomenon. Later she heard talking as well, which became
> unpleasant in character. Finally she appeared at her niece's home at 2 a.m.
> claiming that she had received spoken orders for doing so. Her hallucinosis
> continued following admission to hospital, but there were no other psychotic
> experiences or beliefs. Her symptoms responded rapidly to treatment with a
> phenothiazine drug. She agreed to move from her lonely surroundings into a
> residential home, where she remained symptom-free and mentally alert up to
> time of writing (3 years) even after all treatment had been discontinued. She
> gained and retained complete "insight".

In my experience, auditory hallucinosis of the deaf is usually abolished
by relatively small doses of so-called tranquillising drugs.

Blindness and especially severely impaired vision are not infrequently associated with visual illusions and true hallucinations.
Bartlett (1951) reviewed the literature, and found that the majority of
patients (including his own case) recognised the imaginary nature of
their experiences, and tended to assume an amused attitude towards
them. Occasionally, a patient showed no or variable "insight",
possibly because he was dementing. The way in which a hallucinosis

of this type may become interwoven with paranoid symptoms and personality factors was demonstrated in the following case:

> Mr. T.W., a widower aged 79, had been a meticulous and reserved man, supposedly of Victorian outlook. He had risen to the higher ranks of the Civil Service. His marriage took place after a ten years' courtship, and had been characterised by few sexual activities and childlessness. Following his wife's death, he allowed a nephew and his family to live in his house, with the understanding that they would look after him. In spite of treatment, bilateral glaucoma had led to gradual blindness over the preceding six years. Finally, the patient was only able to distinguish light and dark. Even before this stage had been reached, he had begun to be visually hallucinated. At first he realised that his experiences were the result of his eye condition, but later on he thought they were real while they occurred, though admitting to some doubts later. He would see complex scenes mainly featuring athletic young men stripped to the waist, and green in colour. No women ever appeared; only animals with large open mouths. Later he reported that the men were able to read his thoughts and put poisoned powders in his drink. His hallucinosis and schizophrenic thought content failed to respond to chlorpromazine and related drugs.

It is of interest, but in view of the content of his hallucinosis not surprising, that narcoanalytic exploration revealed homosexual orientation and experience in the patient's early adult life. Initially, there was no evidence of intellectual impairment, and his high intelligence level was confirmed by tests. However, over the subsequent four years he rapidly demented. When last investigated, he tended to become severely confused at night, but probably was no longer hallucinated. In my experience, the hallucinoses of the recently blind —in contrast to the paranoid psychoses of the deaf—do not respond to phenothiazine drugs, possibly because they are more neurological in character; Bartlett (1951) compared the hallucinoses of the blind to the phenomenon of phantom-limb.

Organic paranoid symptoms are very commonly encountered in acute confusional states. When patients are severely disturbed, and level of awareness as well as degree of orientation cannot be easily defined, the true nature of the psychosis may not be recognised. Patients of this type will almost certainly be admitted to a psychiatric unit, where observation will reveal the fluctuating nature of the confusion and of the paranoid symptoms, which moreover tend to be variable and poorly systematised. The sudden onset of persecutory behaviour in elderly people should always suggest the presence of an acute delirious reaction with an underlying physical disorder, which might quickly respond to treatment in a medical or surgical department.

Paranoid symptoms and schizophrenia-like features in patients with chronic brain syndromes, e.g. in senile dementia, are also variable and evanescent. Often they can be directly derived from the memory defect; delusions of theft in old people, who hoard and hide their belongings and then forget where, are the commonest example. A little more complex, in terms of underlying psychopathology, are fleeting delusions of jealousy concerning the behaviour of the aged spouse, and sometimes dangerously aggressive episodes with subsequent amnesia. The way in which paranoid symptomatology of dementia is shaped by personality traits, as well as its transitory nature, were illustrated by a case record in chapter III (Mr. S., p.68). Occasionally, complex and puzzling symptomatology may be due to a hidden cerebro-arteriosclerotic process:

> Mr. We. had been a healthy and happy man without any family history of mental disorder. Originally a motor mechanic and taxi driver, he retired at the age of 46 after receiving a considerable legacy. In his fifties he began to live with a friend's widow; he also belonged to a masonic lodge, various social clubs, and engaged in numerous hobbies. His illness started at the age of 63, after an abdominal operation, belated marriage to his mistress, and dissatisfaction over the purchase of a house. He became sleepless and agitated. A leading psychiatrist diagnosed depression and treated him with ECT. After a good initial response, he became pathologically elated. He began to threaten his wife and to allege that she had defrauded him of £30,000. A year after the onset of symptoms, he presented as a rather puzzled-looking man, jocular in manner but at the same time self-reproachful and sleepless. His blood pressure was raised (190/125), and there was generalised hypertonus, his deep reflexes were increased, and his plantar responses were only doubtfully normal. Some difficulties with recent memory were partially confirmed on learning tests. However, his cerebrospinal fluid, and his electro- as well as pneumoencephalograms showed no definite abnormalities. He was again treated with ECT, as the diagnosis was thought to be one of a mixed manic-depressive state. Treatment had to be abandoned, as he became euphoric and unduly confused. His ideas, that his wife had defrauded him (the sum having risen to £50,000), and that she was trying to keep him in hospital, became more prominent. Phenothiazine therapy produced no real change. He developed an odd manneristic gait, and at a conference of the senior staff a diagnosis of catatonic schizophrenia was suggested. After a period at home and attendance at an occupational centre, he had to be admitted to another hospital. After a few weeks (three years after the onset of symptoms) he developed aphasia and right-sided hemiplegia, dying a month later.

This patient's unusual case has been quoted at some length, because it illustrates two points: Polymorphous psychopathology, i.e. the successive appearance of depressive, hypomanic and paranoid symptoms in the presence of doubtful physical and psychological evidence of brain changes, should always raise suspicion of an organic psychosis. Secondly, a diagnosis of late catatonic schizophrenia is hardly ever correct in elderly persons. In them, odd disturbances of gait, and tic-like manneristic movement are almost always due to cerebral organic changes.

(4) *Functional paranoid psychoses* form a group of illnesses characterised by paranoid and schizophrenic symptoms in the setting of a personality which is not at all, or only very minimally, affected by senile or arteriosclerotic changes. The extent to which the patient's personality becomes involved in schizophrenic modes of experiencing and thinking varies from case to case, and it would take up too much space if we were to illustrate this by clinical records. The reader will, in any case, be familiar with identical pictures presented by younger patients, whose illnesses have been labelled as paranoia, paraphrenia or paranoid schizophrenia.

The mildest illnesses in this graduated series are often symptomatologically indistinguishable from paranoid personality reactions, except that they are much less modifiable by social measures. The patients may, most characteristically, suffer from paranoid beliefs concerning their neighbours; they feel themselves envied and spied upon, remarks are misinterpreted, or patients may even think they overhear conversations emanating from next door or upstairs. Usually these experiences are limited to the patient's home and may not recur for some time, following a change of domicile. Next in degree of severity are patients who, in addition, experience various more bizarre types of interference; smells and gases are directed at them, rays are shone, or photographs are taken, usually in embarrassing situations and with ill-concealed sexual significance. Finally, patients may exhibit so-called process symptoms: telepathic experiences of various kinds (a South African bishop showed his continuing, wholly imaginary, attachment to a former parishioner in England by pulling on her right leg at night!); passivity feelings (a patient spasmodically spun round due to the sun's influence); interference with thinking; being subjected to a running commentary of voices discussing the patient in the third person. Extraordinary experiences may be lived through in phantastic scenes: the patient is taking part in a television programme, is experimented on by students in a medical school, sees and converses with the Archangel Gabriel, to quote only a few examples of what in the past has been called paraphrenia phantastica. As a rule, patients continue to function quite well in the areas of self-care and domestic activities. Many are never seen by psychiatrists, but in others disorders of behaviour make admission to mental hospital necessary, where symptoms continue, in the great majority of cases.

(5) *Affective admixtures* complicate the picture in a large proportion of patients (in 50 of 72 in my consecutive sample). Ecstasy and elation are far less common at this age than anxiety and depression, which are almost always entirely congruous with the content of the psychotic experiences. One is often tempted to surmise that the patients are simply frightened and distressed by their paranoid symptoms, but often schizophrenic and affective symptoms wax and wane (especially following treatment) independently of one another, and the patient is clearly exhibiting both types of reaction simultaneously or consecutively. This was also pointed out by Janzarik (1957) who expressed regret that the unitary concept of psychosis (*Einheitspsychose*) is no longer current. Instead, we tend to speak of schizo-affective illnesses, implying that both types of mental reaction are present, one influencing the other. At the same time, making a correct differential diagnosis has now become a matter of practical importance, if we assume that schizophrenic and affective symptoms respond to different therapeutic agents. It is often taught that paranoid symptomatology, and even "process symptoms" such as influence and passivity experiences, may be regarded as forming part of an affective illness, as long as they can be shown to arise from the patient's feelings of inferiority, badness and guilt, and do not derive from a position of imagined superiority. Following this rule, the original diagnosis of affective psychosis had to be changed to one of schizophrenia in only three of 100 depressive patients, though about 40 had shown some paranoid or schizophreniform symptoms at the time of admission (Post, 1962b). However, in patients with marked paranoid symptoms, but little obvious depression, I frequently fail to make the correct choice of treatment:

Mr. T. was described as a shy and withdrawn man, who had been a nervous child, much teased on account of a slight speech defect, and given to sleep-walking. He had worked in the same firm for 44 years. He did not marry until the age of 37, and remained a widower following his wife's death a few years later. With his small daughter, he returned to the family home. At the age of 58, he attended a psychiatric out-patient department with depression, vague delusions of bodily disorder and ideas of reference, including the belief that he gave off unpleasant odours. The symptoms were so vague, that it was impossible to find out whether he ever lost them again. Four years later, he became very quiet and withdrawn; he drew out all his savings, "in case anything happens to me", but then felt suddenly that faked notes had been planted on him by the police. He began to think that the house was watched and that his conversations were recorded. The sister with whom he was living became seriously depressed, and he shared her delusion of imminent eviction. Both started to remove their belongings from the house, and this led to the sister's admission to our care. She responded well to treatment and the brother's condition came to the psychiatric social worker's notice. Finally, he agreed to his own admission.

Under observation, he was only mildly subdued, but gave the impression of being at times auditorily hallucinated. He developed no fresh delusions in the hospital setting, but remained convinced of the reality of past persecutions. A tentative diagnosis of schizophrenia was made. On high dosage treatment with a phenothiazine drug, trifluoperazine, he appeared to gain insight into the pathological nature of his past ideas, which did not recur on his return home. However, he soon ceased attending the out-patient clinic, and refused to admit the PSW to his home. The patient's daughter found him suspicious and withdrawn, but there was no return of overt symptoms for some eighteen months. He was readmitted, because he ate and slept poorly, and heard noises in the night. He thought that people from upstairs entered his flat and left dud banknotes about. They seemed to drug him, because he would go off to sleep suddenly. In hospital, he was restless in an odd and rather manneristic fashion, and admitted that he frequently heard mumbling voices. This time it was decided to treat him with an allegedly anti-depressive drug, imipramine. Again he lost his symptoms and called them, in retrospect, "imaginary". He continued his rather withdrawn existence at home, soon stopping out-patient attendances and tablets. After six weeks, he became lethargic, neglected himself and appeared suspicious. His family doctor made him resume imipramine, with good therapeutic effect. When seen a few weeks later, he described how he had again become fully convinced that people planted faked notes on him, and described with insight how he had thought he was drugged because he slept very heavily and used to wake with a funny taste in his mouth.

This case has been described at length because it is typical of a large number of patients with chronic mental illnesses without intellectual deterioration (Mr. T. showed no cognitive changes after eight years), but characterised by a mixture of affective and schizophrenic symptoms. Equally good response achieved in these patients with so-called anti-depressive and anti-schizophrenic treatments underlines our ignorance of the nosological status and true nature of affective and schizophrenic illnesses in late life, as well as of their response to drug therapies.

AETIOLOGY AND PROGNOSIS

While we have no knowledge of the basic causes of schizophrenia at any age, a number of constitutional, personality and social features are said to be encountered unduly often in elderly people diagnosed as suffering from this disorder (in the widest sense of the word).

The genetic-hereditary aspects of "late paraphrenia" have been extensively discussed by Kay and Roth (1961). Here we will only refer to their main conclusions. In their English and Swedish material, these workers found the risk among patients' children and siblings of developing schizophrenia to be far lower than that generally given for younger schizophrenic probands. On the other hand, eight first-degree relatives of 99 late paraphrenics had developed paranoid psychoses late in life, as against only two of some 200 elderly depressives. Some hereditary predisposition to late life schizophrenia appeared to exist. In addition, Kay & Roth suggested that genetic influences may manifest themselves throughout the patients' lives by favouring the development of certain personality features. Jealousy, suspiciousness, arrogance, eccentricity, emotional coldness and extreme solitariness (i.e. paranoid and schizoid traits) were found in the previous personalities of 45 per cent of cases. In addition, many were unduly sensitive and explosive in temperament, had belonged to minority religious sects, or had shown sexual inadequacies and deviations. Related to these traits were frequent failure to marry (even after the birth of illegitimate children), delay of marriage and small number of children. It was not surprising that these patients tended to be much more frequently socially isolated than elderly people with affective illnesses. Like other workers, Kay and Roth found that deafness was unduly often associated with late paraphrenia. On the other hand, Janzarik (1957) stressed that most of his patients had a pyknic habitus, and had been capable people, who had continued to work long past the age of official retirement. He remarked that the proportion of single persons was much lower than that found in young schizophrenics, and this accords with my own experience. Hirschmann and Klages (1957) reported similar observations concerning body-build and temperament, but like Kay and Roth, they also found that the human relationships of their patients had often been faulty. Half of them had never married, and others had no children on account of late age at marriage. Many were judged to show physical stigmata of an "inter-sex type". No attempts have so far been made to link specific constitutional, personality and social features to types of symptomatology. At present, all we can say is that a considerable proportion of late life schizophrenics have shown good adjustment to the demands and stresses of life, at any rate on the surface.

Many writers have pointed out that the outcome of schizophrenia in late life was relatively favourable. Patients did not suffer personality deterioration; volitional changes and affective incongruity were rarely seen. Outside the area of paranoid experiencing, patients might continue to function efficiently in a socially tolerant environment. Many patients never came to psychiatric attention; on the other hand, those who finally required mental hospital admission were rarely discharged. This was confirmed by Kay and Roth (1961), who found that remissions obtained by the use of ECT and of tranquillising drugs (up to 1955) were almost always temporary. Some of their patients eventually showed affective blunting or incongruity, with loss of active paranoid delusions. They admitted, however, that in infirm and often deaf old people these changes might be difficult to distinguish from those of genuine organic dementia. Cerebrol-arteriosclerotic or senile changes supervened in 21 per cent, probably not more frequently than in a sample of the non-psychiatric elderly population.

My recent personal experiences of treating schizophrenics are limited to patients willing to enter hospital. These patients may be unrepresentative of the ordinary run of paranoid cases, and few of them required long-term mental hospital care. All the same, over two-thirds of this consecutive sample of elderly paranoid people exhibited "process-symptoms" of schizophrenia. The more recently admitted patients were all treated with adequate courses of so-called psychotropic drugs, mainly trifluoperazine. Some patients, chosen at random, were initially given placebo tablets, but none of them improved on independent "blind" assessment. After a six weeks' course on the drug, only 4 of 25 patients had failed to show some degree of improvement. More prolonged treatment resulted in the complete remission of schizophrenic symptoms in 27 of 35 patients. (For a fuller account of these preliminary results see Post, 1962). At the time of writing, 51 patients have been followed over three years.

5

In none had schizophrenic or paranoid symptoms been present before the age of 50, and in most they had begun to appear during the seventh decade of life. Twenty-eight patients had full courses of a psychotropic (phenothiazine) drug; 23, mostly treated during a somewhat earlier period, had not received any or only inadequate drug treatment. Sixteen of the 23 inadequately treated patients continued to exhibit marked mental symptoms throughout the whole of the follow-up period, and only 4 had lasting remissions. By contrast, adequate treatment failed completely in only 3 of 28 patients, and over one-half ultimately responded lastingly to psychotropic preparations. A small number suffered psychotic symptoms over lengthy periods, usually because they had, from time to time, failed to continue treatment.

The results of drug therapy are perhaps not quite so impressive when we assess patients not only for the presence of florid psychotic phenomena, but also for occasional mild symptoms and continuing paranoid attitudes. All the same, only 8 of the 28 fully treated patients showed continuous mild symptoms over three years, as compared with 20 of the 23 untreated cases. Complete retrospective realisation of the pathological nature of their past experiences was achieved by only 8 people belonging to the treated group; the rest remained convinced of the reality of past persecutions, or wavered in their views.

A statistical analysis of data will be carried out when all patients in this consecutive series have been followed through three years, but the figures as they stand at present suggest very strongly that the treatment and prognosis of elderly paranoid patients (at any rate of those willing to come for help) has been revolutionised thanks to modern drugs, provided always they are used adequately. We may add that there have been so far only six patients whose symptoms did not recur when phenothiazines were discontinued. The remainder either failed to remit completely, or more often relapsed as soon as the dosage was allowed to drop below maintenance level, or the tablets were discontinued. So, in the majority of patients in this sample, maintenance therapy, usually at a very low level, may be required indefinitely. It will be some years before the long-term results of modern drug treatment of schizophrenia can be assessed. To date, my impression is that they are likely to be very much better in elderly paranoid patients than in young schizophrenics, whose personalities are usually much more extensively affected by the disease.

CHAPTER VI

PERSONALITY DISORDERS IN OLD AGE

DEFINITIONS

The three preceding chapters dealt with definite mental illnesses. According to K. Schneider (1955) and his school, deviations seen in these disorders, i.e. in the psychoses, cannot be plotted at the extreme ends of a continuous normal distribution curve, as can be done in the case of non-psychotic abnormalities of psychological functioning. Psychotic ways of experiencing, thinking and behaving are held to be phenomena entirely different from those seen in patients with minor psychological disorders. Basic to this way of psychiatric thinking is an analogy with what is said to hold in the field of intellectual subnormality; most mentally subnormal people are found at the lower end of the normal distribution curve of intelligence test scores, but there is also a much smaller group of what used to be called imbeciles and idiots, whose intellectual defects are due to some definite pathology, such as faulty cerebral development, brain injury or metabolic abnormalities. In the Schneiderian view the psychoses, even the functional ones, are also assumed to be caused by some somatic abnormality. They are therefore looked upon as definite illnesses, and contrasted with disabling conditions of varying severity which present only quantitative variations of modes of psychological functioning, common to all human beings. In other words, persons with character disorders, psychopathic personalities, or psycho-neuroses are held to vary excessively from the statistical norm in such universal traits as acquisitiveness, aggressiveness, sexual drives and aims, ritualistic warding off, capacity of denial and dissociation, etc.

While not fully subscribing to this theory, I have found it convenient to deal in this book with organic, affective and schizophrenic psychoses separately from milder conditions, such as character disorders, personality changes and neuroses. We may remind ourselves that in senile dementia, the organic psychosis which is closest to normal ageing, psychological investigators were able to demonstrate that the psychometric pattern was very different from that seen in the normal and orderly decline of mental abilities with age. This indicated that senile dementia was due to a pathological process, and not just the result of premature or accelerated ageing; that it was an illness, rather than a condition at the extreme end of a graded continuum (Chapter III). This sharp distinction between illness and excessive reaction to stress is much more difficult to maintain in the case of some melancholic and some schizophrenic psychoses, in which we often find the disorder to be limited in extent, and understandable in terms of the patient's personality and life situation. Moreover, some of these conditions respond well to manipulating the patient's social conditions. Perhaps we are dealing here with people of neurotic make-up or with personality weaknesses who, under severe stress, break down not just with an exacerbation of lifelong personality deviations, but with mental "illnesses" (in the Schneiderian sense).

Personality disorders are characterised by undue preponderance or deficiency of certain features in the personality structure. This may present a disability to the person himself, or may largely be a problem to others. In the first category are excessive introversion, social withdrawal, suspiciousness, a depressive temperament, excessive fatiguability, lack of drive and of sexual interests. In the second category, we may name excessive extroversion, aggressiveness, acquisitiveness or sex-drive (often with deviant aims). Personality deviations of any type lead to impaired relations with others, but an excess of outgoing tendencies, especially in the presence of strong aggressive, acquisitive, or sexual components, may lead to unrestrained "acting-out" of these drives, and present a greater social problem. Such *character disorders* or *psychopathic personalities* may be present throughout life. Some, however, may become less troublesome with increasing age, while others may assume disabling proportions in late life only, and are then referred to as *senile personality changes* or *senile character disorders*. People with certain personality deficiencies may also suffer from *psychoneuroses*, which are usually regarded as ways of dealing with (external) stresses and (internal) presses. Psychoneurotic symptoms fall into a number of well-structured patterns, which may be interpreted as presenting more or less successful ways of avoiding anxiety. In phobic states, anxiety is said to be displaced to certain situations—some of them inside the body (certain types of hypochondriasis). In hysteria, there is conversion of the painful affect into psychical or physical defects, often resulting in some doubtful "gain" (e.g. removal from the source of anxiety). Obsessional symptomatology may be interpreted as warding off, and as symbolic removal of anxiety.

In practice, individuals tend to exhibit mixtures of all these "non-psychotic" behaviour patterns, but certain combinations are more common than others. Excessive extroverted trends with strong aggressiveness and acquisitiveness make for acting-out behaviour, rather than for symbolic solution of problems by the formation of phobic or obsessional symptoms; such persons, not infrequently, also exhibit hysterical mechanisms. By contrast, unduly introverted, timid, sensitive, anxious, or depressive persons hardly ever act out, but in them the occurrence of obsessional and phobic symptomatology is more common.

Psychiatric readers will be familiar with these speculations on the relationship between personality and neurosis, on the symbolic and psycho-dynamic significance of neurotic symptoms, on psychopathy, and on the concept of acting-out behaviour. These matters have been re-ventilated here, because they help us to understand the special features of minor psychiatric disorders in late life. We saw (Chapter I) that certain changes of personality structure with age have been well documented: increasing turning inward, withdrawal into the inner circle of the family, and diminution of emotionally directed outward drives. We shall therefore expect all forms of acting-out and psycho-pathic behaviour, as well as tendencies to the formation of hysterical conversion symptoms to become increasingly unusual with rising age. On the other hand, it will not surprise us to find that dysthymic, sensitive, and restrictive personality traits, as well as a tendency to phobic and obsessive symptom formation will not diminish, but may even become more marked. We shall see that this prediction of the way in which ageing is likely to modify, or produce minor psycho-logical disturbances, is broadly correct.

ABNORMAL PERSONALITIES

What is the influence of ageing on personality disorders which manifest themselves in childhood, adolescence or early adult life? This question cannot be answered unequivocally, as there are no follow-up studies of cohorts of disturbed younger persons into late life. All we can say is that in the psychiatric clinic we seldom diagnose elderly patients as suffering from psychopathic personality, behaviour disorder, or severe character neurosis. Related to this is the frequently documented and very striking decrease in the crime rate with increasing age. This trend is slightly modified in the oldest age group, due to a relative increase of sexual offences, embezzlement and offences against laws regulating the use of drugs and narcotics. These are criminal activities which require little physical strength and agility, and which in some instances may well be symptoms of senile mental changes (for details see Norwood East, 1944, and Jones and Kaplan, 1956). The suggestion has often been made that people with a tendency to aggressive and impulsive behaviour disorders stabilise with increasing age, in that these conditions had been due to delayed psychic maturation. Reference is also made to the dying down of the "storm and stress" of earlier life. Clinical experience certainly favours these views. On the other hand, inquiries into the background of elderly tramps and down-and-outs, usually bring to light lifelong personality defects leading to social failure. Occasionally, it is possible to demonstrate that psychopathic tendencies may continue with undiminished intensity into old age:

Mr. D. came from a good middle-class family, but while still at school began to cause his parents serious concern on account of undisciplined and mildly delinquent behaviour. His short military career in World War I culminated in a cleverly engineered medical discharge. The gifted young man passed easily through the university, and then went on to train for the Church of England. He became engaged to the daughter of a high ecclesiastic dignitary, but shortly before his ordination and marriage he disappeared. He became a Roman Catholic convert and entered a seminary in preparation for the priesthood. After a while he was discovered in compromising situations with young lads. Punitive transfers to stricter institutions had no effect, and he was finally summoned before a specially convened ecclesiastical court. He permitted its proceedings to go on for quite a while before placing himself outside the jurisdiction of the court by announcing, for once truthfully, that he had got married.

The lady in question afterwards admitted that she realised how unstable and unreliable her husband was, but she found his personality irresistible, and later on forgave him many infidelities. She remained the main breadwinner of the marriage, and had to support both daughters through illegitimate pregnancies and related happenings. The patient himself kept himself more or less above water by doing stage work and minor artistic jobs. During the Second World War he found a niche in the Temporary Civil Service. At a later date he earned not inconsiderable sums of money by entertaining London theatre queues, and also by striking up acquaintanceships with a number of artistes, whom he used as cover for minor confidence tricks. Finally, at the age of 68, he began to suffer from quite severe attacks of depression and mania, which required several admissions to hospital. Contact with him was maintained during the intervening periods, when he continued his previous activities. His lack of restraint and sense of decorum was illustrated by the way in which he related his many, and always completely unsuccessful attempts, at making amorous advances to young female foreign visitors, whom he would accompany on long train journeys to distant suburbs.

This section may be summarised as follows: In spite of the absence of systematic long-term studies, a strong impression persists that the severity of psychopathic disorders diminishes with rising age in the great majority of cases. Certainly, advice is sought for these conditions only when mental illness or deterioration become superadded, or when withdrawal of social support through bereavement or moving away of other members of the family makes permanent care necessary.

SENILE CHARACTER DISORDERS

These can always be traced back to slight personality defects which had not given rise to obvious difficulties earlier in life, but which have become more prominent and troublesome in old age. The way in which the later personality may be turned into a caricature of the earlier one is illustrated by the following case record:

Mrs. I., aged 84, had risen from working class origins into the small business class. Both her sister and her surviving son had had treatment for depressive illnesses. This son had remained unmarried, and had continued to live with his mother after she had been widowed for a second time. Nothing reliable could be ascertained about her marital adjustment, but she had always shown certain mild personality defects, which had not interfered with her being an excellent worker, housewife, and mother. Within the family she was overpossessive; outside she was shy and timid. She seemed to dislike close relationships, would become suspicious, easily take offence, and her few friendships would tend to "sour up", to use the son's eloquent phrase. She was always inclined to look on the black side of things, and when crossed would become tearful and describe herself as a poor little woman. She might even develop headaches or retire to bed for a day or two. After her second son's death on active service, she for a time attended spiritualist meetings. At the age of 73, and after yet another failure in maintaining a friendship, she suddenly began to complain of getting old and to take tremendous care of herself. During the winter months she would never leave her home, and at the threat of fog she would take to her bed, claiming that she had bronchitis and asthma. The slightest ailment, e.g. a nose bleed, would throw her into a panic. Her son's attempts to go out in the evening usually provoked dramatic scenes and recriminations. In an attempt to give the patient more social support, mother and son moved next door to her sister, who was, however, soon accused of subverting the son's affections and of stealing. On at least one occasion, bank notes to the value of £50 were found hidden all over the patient's room. Physically she was found to be healthy; orientation and memory were outstandingly good, and even psychological testing failed to bring to light any defects of cognitive functioning.

In this and similar patients, who as a rule show some intellectual deterioration as well, the character disorder is best understood as an exaggeration of the normal "turning inward" of people as they grow old. Senile character changes tend to become a serious problem only in persons with lifelong poorly developed outgoing tendencies. In them, relationships with other persons become even more restricted, possessive and unpleasurable. Earlier difficulties in adjusting to others in an easy give-and-take lead to a rigid outlook and haughty isolation. The world has always been looked upon as full of hidden dangers, and now it is regarded as downright hostile. The future was seen in the past as uncertain and threatening; now a gloomy, worrying and anxious outlook becomes habitual; careful attention to bodily health increases to hypochondriasis, proclivity to "saving for a rainy day" and habitual frugality turn into miserliness.

In *senile recluses*, social withdrawal and turning into oneself are most strikingly exemplified. Sheldon (1948) and other general medical writers have described these lonely eccentrics (4 per cent of Sheldon's sample of elderly people living in their own homes) as particularly vigorous and apparently happy old people. They contrasted them with persons who had become isolated through strokes of fate (Miller, 1963). However, the conditions in which many people living in voluntary isolation are eventually discovered make one wonder whether odd ideas and beliefs may not have been hidden behind the rugged facade. This is another group of elderly persons which has never been studied systematically, but Granick and Zeman (1960) carried out an analysis of newspaper cuttings referring to 105 recluses. Their sample was, no doubt, biased by the sensational way in which subjects had come to public notice, but a few interesting findings emerged. Women had become recluses as frequently as men, and the process had probably started early in life, as 42 per cent had never married. Sometimes the hermit-like existence had been shared with a sibling. The recluses usually lived in apparently poverty-stricken and neglected circumstances, but most of them were comfortably off or even rich. Often, they measured up to the popular stereotype of the miserly recluse, in that large sums of money had been hoarded and hidden in the home.

Other *severe forms of senile personality change* are also not very common. Albrecht (1951) found that only 11 per cent of a representative sample of elderly people stood out from the rest on account of the following characteristics: they were described as cantankerous, irascible, self-centred and unable to get along with others. They did not enjoy people, or social and recreational activities. They were unhappy and lived from day to day. Their interests were entirely centred in the past, and they met problems in a childish and impulsive manner. They vegetated, and did nothing, even though their physical condition did not prohibit activity. Finally, they gave little attention to their appearance.

More commonly senile changes affect mainly areas of personality functioning, such as sleep, appetite, sex-drive, etc. which may be regarded as *psychosomatic*. These have been studied by a number of authors and related to numerous problems of old age, over and above those arising from the accentuation of earlier potentially disabling personality traits. Berner and Hoff (1959) have sought to demonstrate how some crises occurring during the process of ageing might be understood in terms of existentialist philosophy; a stage is reached in life when people realise (Camus' *Awakening*) that, sooner or later, there will no longer be any future left to them. This ought to lead to a greater appreciation of the present; of existing, as contrasted with a concern with future-centred, achieving. When this realisation is suppressed or repressed, it will be forced upon the individual towards the end of his life, when he no longer has the same resilient capacity for readjustment. He may then be unable to relinquish the need to achieve something, and feel that he has not yet completed his life task. He has failed to learn to enjoy existing in the present, and in present relationships with others. Berner and Hoff also point out that loss of the future dimension is better tolerated by people who remain secure in the role they have played throughout adult life, and who feel that they continue to be accepted in that role. Realisation that since their youth there has been considerable devaluation of the status and role of the aged may prove critical in some persons. We need not here recapitulate the importance allotted to role-playing and communication by certain schools of social psychiatry, which are related to the existentialist point of view.

In a more down-to-earth fashion, Mead (1962) pointed out that many personality changes can be understood and better tolerated when it is realised that they arise from the inability (for realistic reasons) of old people to gain satisfaction in planning the future. Satisfaction tends to be sought in the moment, by using various denial mechanisms. One of them he calls the syndrome of "grasping at straws", as shown by sudden out-of-character interests, unusual health fads, and religious affiliations. In the "lack of acceptance" syndrome, there is denial of physical disabilities and a tendency to overdo things, especially as regards physical exercise. Hypochondriasis may not be very different in origin, i.e. failure to accept slight physical defects. The tendency of old people to complain about or to ignore physical symptoms due to minor disorders was investigated by Kahn *et al.* (1958). The number of complaints was found to be independent of the actual medical status, sex and degree of mental preservation of a person. Somatic complaining was a feature mainly of people with limited resources of coping with the environment, to the extent that complaining seemed to be their principal mode of adaptation. Most people who denied illness which was actually present showed evidence of diffuse cerebral dysfunction, much as is found in anosognosia associated with more specific defects.

Returning to psychosomatic dysfunctions, it is usually said that old people not only require less *sleep*, or tend to take cat-naps during the day, but also that they often sleep badly at night. However, Ginzberg (1955) reported that sleep disturbances were found, depending on the method of ascertainment employed, in only 10 to 20 per cent of elderly subjects. They were equally uncommon in residents of a county home (i.e. public institution) as in inmates of a psychiatric unit. The presence of sleep disorders was not related to a higher age or the presence of chronic organic brain-changes. On the contrary, it was more frequent in the less deteriorated subjects, and significantly associated with affective disturbances as well as with constipation and poor socialisation (both probably secondary to the affective disorder). Chronic sleeplessness in the elderly should not be looked upon as the inevitable result of damage to some cerebral mechanisms, but rather as a sign of anxiety, depression and maladjustment. Sleep disturbance seen in acute confusional states is, of course, almost always of recent onset.

Similarly, *digestive difficulties* should never be regarded as due to old age itself (Savitsky, 1953). For instance, it just is not true that old people have an aversion for meat; this was found in only six per cent of Sheldon's (1948) sample. The role of mastication, especially the absence or ill-fit of dentures, in causing digestive disorders and feeding problems has probably been exaggerated, as most foods can be satisfactorily chewed by the gums. Old people who cannot tolerate dentures have often had difficulties in adapting to any new situation in the past, and have always had food prejudices. (Persistent complaints about new dentures are occasionally the outstanding symptom of depressive illness.) Comparison of young and old groups has shown that constipation is not characteristic of old age either. Elderly people who are constipated tended to have had the same complaints and preoccupations when they were younger. Increased bowel-consciousness occurs with rising age, and is related to a general rise in hypochondriacal concerns. Savitsky also concedes that poor adaptation to the stresses of old age generates anxiety, which may lead to digestive symptoms and feeding problems in people with earlier prejudices and aversions. He further suggests that the nature of the emotional problems can sometimes be suspected from the kinds of foods rejected or demanded, in that they appear to have symbolic, almost magical, significance: milk, milk products and slops are security foods; chocolate, sweets, ice cream, etc. are reward foods; red meat, chicken, eggs are often believed to restore health and energy, and may be regarded as fetish foods.

Addictions may be briefly mentioned here. In keeping with the resourcefulness required in their pursuit, they do not present a frequent problem in geriatrics. Habituation to sleeping draughts and sedatives is, of course, very common, but as the causative pain and distress may be due to chronic and incurable physical and psychological conditions, excessive use of drugs (provided it is supervised) may be the lesser of many evils. To judge from histories obtained in elderly psychiatric patients, addictions especially to alcohol in earlier adult life, not infrequently disappear in the late forties or fifties. Fresh addiction to alcohol is occasionally seen in old age. Elderly alcoholics appear to be more often prepared to go through courses of treatment than younger ones, and the results, whichever method used, have in my experience been gratifying. However, the number of cases treated and followed up does not permit any conclusions as to the permanency of the cures effected.

Just as was the case with sexual ageing (Chapter I), there is no precise information available on *sexual disorders* of elderly people, apart from some criminal statistics. A number of authors have attempted to generalise on the basis of psychological and clinical impressions (for summaries see Jones and Kaplan, 1956, and Cameron, 1956). We saw in previous chapters that the content of the illness in patients with late schizophrenia is often of a sexual nature. This is also found, to a smaller extent, with affective and organic psychoses. It usually reflects overt or latent sexual abnormalities in earlier life, and is rarely seen in patients who up to the time of their mental illness had had no sexual problems. Contrary to expectation, decreasing libido and impotence only rarely figure as preoccupations or obvious precipitants in the milder psychiatric disorders of elderly people. In men, sudden cessation of sexual interests and activities is almost always a symptom of psychiatric illness, especially of depression. Women who, following gynaecological operations, refuse to resume sexual relations or who claim to have reached a sexual age limit have almost always been frigid and resentful of physical approaches for some time previously, and in relation to long-standing marital maladjustment.

What little we know about *sexual deviations* in old age all concerns men. The old idea that sexual misdemeanours of old men are the unfortunate results of diminished control in early senile dementia is now regarded as an over-simplification of a complex situation. In actual fact, senile cognitive changes are usually conspicuous by their absence in elderly men charged with sexual offences, though some-times long-practising homosexuals are caught because they have become careless in covering up their activities. Hirschmann (1962) observed a group of aged sexual offenders, and found that almost all offences were committed against children, ranging from exhibitionism to activities in one way or other falling short of coitus. He pointed out that, normally, sexual union is only attempted after increasing personal contact, involving attraction, courtship and love. Elderly men are likely to suffer frequent failure in these preliminaries, and may, moreover, be capable only of partial sexual acts, which are not acceptable to younger women. On the other hand, children tend to be friendly, submissive, inquisitive, and often not unfamiliar with partial sexual activities, like masturbation. Once an old man has achieved satisfaction, the acts are likely to be repeated, and unlikely to stop on account of threats or actual punishments. Hirschmann reports that most men in his group had no previous records of sexual perversions or delinquencies, but that a proportion had always had problems of various kinds in the sexual field. Often they were men who had valued themselves almost exclusively in terms of their ability to achieve successful sexual intercourse. If they were unable to sublimate their libido, when intercourse with women became difficult or impossible, they tended to seek activities with children. They usually presented other personality changes as well, but successful psycho-therapeutic management was sometimes possible.

PSYCHONEUROSES

Elderly patients suffering only from neurotic symptoms are infrequently seen in psychiatric clinics. Kessel and Shepherd (1962) found that in the statistics of psychiatric hospitals and out-patient clinics, the proportion of cases labelled "neurosis" reached its peak around the age of 30, and fell sharply with rising age. By contrast, the prevalence of conditions diagnosed as "neurotic" by family doctors rose steadily up to the age of 35–45, and then remained at about the same level well beyond the age of 65. There appear to be only two, not mutually exclusive, explanations for this discrepancy: (1) family physicians refer to psychiatrists fewer and fewer patients as they grow older, (2) they apply the term neurotic in a different way from specialists. Busse and his group (1960, 1961) found among 222 subjects over 60, resident in Durham (North Carolina), only 86 entirely normal persons. Fifty-six were classified as neurotic, 25 of their number to a severe degree. In addition, 42 subjects were regarded as having neurotic as well as mild cerebral-organic disorders.

Pure anxiety states characterised by sweating, trembling, palpi-tating, localised flushing and dilated pupils are hardly ever seen in the elderly. Anxiety, even when it is unassociated with any depressive features, manifests itself by unpleasant somatic sensations, especially flutterings in chest or lower abdomen, hypochondriacal elaborations and restlessness. A diagnosis of conversion hysteria is rarely upheld in this age group. Recently established phobic states are unusual, but do occur. Obsessive compulsive symptoms are the only classical psychoneurotic phenomena seen at all frequently among the elderly, notwithstanding a general impression confirmed by Mueller (1953) that the severity of obsessional symptoms of younger people tended to diminish as they grew older. One of Busse's findings was that over half of neurotic elderly people with mixed depressive-hypochondriacal symptoms had shown a different type of psychoneurotic sympto-matology earlier in life. This is not surprising, if one accepts that neurotic symptoms are a way of dealing with anxiety, and that neurotic persons have a lifelong proneness to excessive anxiety. Its sources change with the situations encountered, and different patterns of neurotic symptoms may be called out as a neurotic person becomes older. The following case record illustrates this point:

Mrs. J. was aged 67 when first seen by me.

Between the ages of 3 and 7, she had suffered from bilious headaches; at the age of 6 she had a severe panic when her photograph was taken, fearing that she would be "stuck in a frame for life." When aged 15, she was shocked by the death of a brother, and when another brother fell ill, she had to keep creeping secretly into his room many times, day and night, to make quite sure that he was still alive.

At the age of 18, she developed fears of heart disease after contact with a case. She had much breathlessness and palpitations, but did a series of amateurish jobs, breaking down, aged 36, in London during the 1917 Zeppelin raids. She spent two months in a resthome where she had psychotherapy.

When aged 38, the patient felt "relieved" by the death of a man, whom she loved but had felt unable to marry, but when aged 42, she did marry a widower after several years of anxiety. He nursed her along, and the marriage was satisfactory. However, aged 44, she spent 4 months in a general hospital with shortness of breath, palpitations and headaches. ("Anxiety State in neurotic personality.")

From 53 to 55, she was seen at the Maudsley Hospital ("Hysteria, mixed") and later on she consulted several eminent psychiatrists.

Between the ages of 55 and 66, the patient had no specific treatment, but often had episodes when she would stay in bed, being worried, anxious and sleepless.

At 67 she received psychotherapy for pains in her arms and chest, and finally she was sent into hospital under my care, because she was getting too depressed; she had much masturbation guilt and ruminated on the possibility of her husband's death.

When aged 67–71, she was supported as an out-patient; she developed fainting turns, but had normal EEGs.

At 72, the patient's husband died, but she felt relatively well, and moved into a boarding house.

At the age of 75, she resumed out-patient attendance; at first she complained about double, triple and quadruple (!) vision, but she did in fact develop permanent diplopia, which a neurologist confirmed to be due to an external rectus palsy, probably produced by pressure of a sclerotic vessel on the 6th cranial nerve.

When aged 76, she had to be readmitted for a few months on account of increasing agitation, importuning and unhappiness.

At 77, the patient attended the out-patient clinic with anxiety feelings associated with unsatisfactory domestic arrangements, and finally,

When aged 79, she obtained an interview with me to seek sympathetic discussion of a blighted romance!

Early in life, anxiety had found expression in this patient directly and psychosomatically; in childhood her symptomatology had been mainly phobic-obsessive; later, the pattern changed to a mixture of anxious and hysterical phenomena. As she entered the involutional or presenile period of life anxious-depressive patterns became established, but hysterical mechanisms were once more evoked under the impact of physical disorders. All these successive waves of psychiatric symptomatology appeared to be caused by life experiences impingeing on an immature, dependent and anxiety-prone personality. Occasionally, one also sees patients whose symptoms remain unchanged throughout life, e.g. a lady of 72 who at the age of 8 ceased to attend school on account of phobias; she was never again able to leave her home unaccompanied, which did not prevent her from marrying and bringing up one (neurotic) daughter.

By far the commonest symptom patterns among the subjects of the North Carolina study were *hypochondriasis* and *depressions*; *fatigue* states, which cannot be explained on an adequate physical basis, are no doubt related to mild affective disorders. In classing these disorders as psychoneuroses, Busse and his associates (1960) used as their criterion that "the psychoneurotic person does not represent a gross distortion of personality." Most of their neurotic elderly subjects suffered from hypochondriasis and depression at the same time; neither was their hypochondriasis bizarre, nor were their depressions associated with delusions of guilt. The concepts of neurotic and masked depression, as well as the relationship of these disorders to hypochondriasis, were fully discussed in Chapter IV. Here we shall only recapitulate very briefly that depressive illnesses in persons with lifelong neurotic propensities tend to be mild; that many elderly people suffer from mild and short depressions, and that hypochondriasis may be the first symptom of more serious depressive illnesses. So, from a theoretical point of view, it is difficult to draw a clear distinguishing line between severe neurosis and mild affective psychosis. On the other hand, longstanding hypochondriasis without obvious depression can usually be traced back to lifelong bodily over-concern; its exaggeration might be interpreted as a character change, rather than as a neurosis in the strict sense of the word.

The sources of anxiety underlying psychoneurotic reactions in old age are obvious and numerous. In contrast to what is found in younger people, sexual problems (e.g. impotence) do not loom large in elderly patients, even when they had been important as aetiological factors in the earlier neurotic disorders. In my experience, conflicts and anxieties arising from relationships with other members of the family are far more important: reactivation of earlier conflicts with children often occurs at a time when roles are reversed. Problems related to dependency and overdependency are frequently encountered. By contrast, anxieties stemming from economic difficulties, physical disease, and interruption of relationships are a common fate borne by many old people without causing psychiatric symptoms. The lot of the aged is often so sad and difficult that the great frequency of minor affective disorders is hardly surprising. As pointed out earlier, classical psychoneurotic syndromes are seen much less frequently than mixtures of anxiety, hypochondriasis and depression.

Hysterical conversion symptoms almost always occur in the setting of other psychiatric illnesses; an amnesic fugue in a depressive patient of inadequate personality, and recurrent attacks of aphonia in a woman who finally turned out to suffer from a severe paranoid-depressive psychosis, are among the cases that come to mind. Diethelm and Rockwell's (1943) contention that, in the elderly, histrionic and infantilistic behaviour were due to emotional reactions, and not dysmnestic-dissociative in origin, has been generally accepted. Disabilities of hearing, sight and memory are often ridiculously exaggerated, but these are now recognised as ways in which depressed, agitated and bewildered old people clamour for help and communicate their distress. In my experience, tics and tic-like motility disorders are the only so-called hysterical symptoms which occur at all frequently in elderly people, without obvious depression or other disorders. A recent case appeared to exemplify the typical situation in which conversion symptoms may occur:

Mrs. L., *aet.* 73, claimed that she had been a normal and outgoing person, and that there had been no mental abnormalities in any members of her family. However, her first husband committed suicide, and she subsequently lived for 20 years with a man who did not marry her. She had little contact with her children and stepchildren. There was an earlier history of numerous operations for relatively minor complaints, but over the last 9 years she had been suffering from severe and widespread osteoarthritis. She was only able to move from bed to wheel-chair. A woman friend of 20 years' standing, by now 80 years old, looked after her extremely well, and shared her house.

Two years previously, the patient had received injection treatments to her joints in a hospital, where she was very happy. Her condition failed to improve, and it was reported that at the threat of being discharged, she began to suffer continuous blinking. After a few days, she discovered that this troublesome condition was relieved by simply keeping her eyes closed. Soon she found she could not open her eyelids, except by pulling them apart. Several ophthalmologists diagnosed her condition as hysterical blepharospasm. She became rather distressed, and was treated at another psychiatric department with anti-depressive drugs and hypnosis, without relief. Her attitude during a stay in our unit was uncomplaining and cheerful. It was thought that occasionally, when believing herself unobserved, she was able to keep her eyes open for a while, and the spasm was definitely absent for about half an hour after awaking in the morning. The psychiatric social worker discovered that the patient's companion had until a few years earlier looked after her own mother, who had been blind for many years before her death. This lady had always taken a great interest in blind people, and had obviously transferred her protective feelings from her mother to the patient. The possibility that our patient, in order to retain her companion, had identified herself with the blind mother was ventilated in some twenty narcoanalytic sessions. But neither this nor hypnotic suggestion and persuasion affected the symptom. The patient refused relief of the assumed anxiety by transfer to long-term nursing care, and reluctantly returned to her home.

In another elderly female patient, odd tic-like mouth spasms appeared to be related to a recent erotic experience. She was treated by a psychotherapist along analytic lines, and the symptom was very greatly improved. In spite of continued attendance at a psychotherapy centre and considerable benefit in relation to a number of emotional problems, this lonely spinster's physical symptoms recurred and persisted. She was observed for nine years, and the suspicion that a small vascular lesion had been the cerebral substrate of her symptoms was strengthened by the occurrence of transitory diplopia, and later of a partial thrombosis of the central retinal artery of one eye, which also showed evidence of a macular haemorrhage. Other elderly patients with tic-like movements have been treated, using behavioural techniques, with equal lack of success. These therapeutic failures, not confined to elderly people, are consistent with a view that tics and similar repetitive, stereotyped movements often have cerebral origin, and that, though much influenced by emotional factors, they are not hysterical symptoms in the accepted sense of the term. But what is hysteria, anyhow?

Phobic symptoms cause disabilities which elderly people and their friends find easy to accept. It is often taken for granted that, with increasing age, people avoid going out on their own and that they do not like to be left alone in the house. Patients are only referred when their symptoms begin to impose unreasonable restrictions on other members of their families, or when a sudden increase of phobic symptoms occurs, usually due to the occurrence of a depressive illness. If the affective disorder can be successfully treated, phobic behaviour almost always returns to its previous manageable level. Occasionally, there is no depression, and the anxiety is entirely related to feelings of insecurity engendered by social changes or pressures, e.g. the threatened departure of a daughter or son following their engagement to be married. Not infrequently, "dizzy" and fainting turns occur in this sort of situation (cerebral causes are not discovered at the time or on follow-up). It is sometimes possible to give patients greater security in a psychotherapeutic relationship, after full physical investigation and reassurance. Often, there are found to exist long-standing personality disorders and associated complex and ambivalent family relationships. It may even be necessary, for the sake of the younger generation, to persuade the old person to accept residential care away from the family.

Obsessional symptoms are quite frequently encountered in our age group, even when the use of the term is restricted by the following characteristics: (1) Repetitive thought content and (not always) behaviour, (2) Attempts at suppressing these phenomena are made, but are ultimately unsuccessful on account of resulting anxiety, (3) The thoughts and actions are recognised by the patient as abnormal (but this last criterion is not accepted as necessarily present by some authorities). Repetitive and reiterative talk, worrying preoccupations and unrelenting hypochondriacal concerns, as well as unpleasant intrusive and recurring thoughts, are found in agitated depressive illnesses, and their clear delimitation from true obsessional phenomena in patients who only express themselves poorly may be impossible in practice. By contrast, perseveration and stereotyped repetitive behaviour seen in organic brain disease bear only superficial resemblance to obsessional symptoms.

Benaim (1956) reviewed 46 patients over 60 with obsessional

phenomena which were sufficiently clear-cut and severe to be included in the final diagnosis. Further experience has amply confirmed his first finding; almost all these patients also exhibited marked affective symptoms, and it is usually true to say that obsessional patients in late life do not come for psychiatric advice unless they are also depressed (a few may have manic episodes, as well). Only 4 patients in Benaim's group appeared to have developed true obsessional symptoms in the setting of an organic psychosis. The remaining patients fell into two groups:

(1) Primarily obsessional patients, with symptoms commencing in childhood, adolescence or early adult life; only 2 of 18 became obsessional after the age of 40. Sexual adjustment had been satisfactory in only two patients of this group, which had a high celibacy rate (44 per cent), and a high incidence of sexual obsessions and of compulsive motor actions.

(2) Primarily affective illnesses with obsessional symptoms occurred in people who had only very rarely experienced obsessional symptoms (as against personality traits) before middle adult life. Solely in association with depressive illnesses, obsessional symptoms appeared for the first time in 16 of 24 patients after the age of 40 (after 60, in nine cases). A larger proportion of these patients claimed good sexual adjustment, and their celibacy rate was lower than that of the first group of primary obsessionals, though still much higher than that of the general population over 60. Symptoms with sexual content and compulsive acts (as against obsessive ruminative symptoms) were much more rarely seen. Primary obsessional symptoms normally improved, and secondary ones often disappeared entirely after the depression remitted. Obsessional symptoms were more likely to persist in patients who had been over 50 years old at the time of their first appearance. Benaim's finding that obsessional phenomena occasionally assume delusional characteristics, and that, in a sense, the patients' frequently expressed fears of "insanity" may come true, has been confirmed (Post, 1962).

The management of disabling obsessional symptoms in elderly people largely resolves itself into treatment of the depressive state with which they are almost always associated. Speculations on the puzzling relationship between obsessions and depression would lead too far. An illustrative case description was given in Chapter IV (Mr. H., pp. 95–6). On account of the unusual symptomatology and the involvement of other members of her family, we shall here quote the case of a lady who developed a chronic obsessional neurosis following a mild depression in her seventieth year:

Mrs. C. was first seen when she was 69 years old. There was nothing unusual about her background, except that she had lost her husband when her only son was three years old. Her grief was severe, and prolonged over several years. Also, she remained overprotective of her son, an anxious and indecisive man. Otherwise she was only a little too meticulous; her personality was warm and affectionate, if rather restricted in outlook. The son, who was approaching the age of 40, had been dithering over an engagement for several years. At last he made definite arrangements to get married. At about this time the patient's brother-in-law died, an event to which she again responded excessively. In this setting, mother and son had a quarrel during which he rebelled against her authority and said several bitter things. The patient developed unpleasant head sensations, sleeplessness and occasional feelings that she would rather be dead. After six months these symptoms subsided, and, when first seen a little later, there was no longer any evidence of depression. Instead, she had developed the fear that she was forgetting what she had read in the newspaper, names of acquaintances, and occurrences in her daily life. She developed an intricate system of checks and counter-checks, in which she involved her son. She half realised that her fears were unreasonable, but became so tense that she had to obtain confirmation of matters she might have forgotten. The patient was followed over eight years, and at no time did there appear any evidence that she was failing in her domestic abilities. Memory tasks were always well performed, and slight patchiness of performance in the area of historical and political dates and names (she was a rather uneducated person) did not get worse. Following the son's marriage, hostility to the daughter-in-law led to serious difficulties, which necessitated intensive psychiatric social work. Finally, the son was helped to move away and to rejoin his wife and children whom he had left, but his guilt and anxiety persisted. At our last contact with the patient, the son was still calling on her every morning and every evening (on his way to and from work) to reassure her over memory "problems" that had accumulated in the meantime. The intensity of the patient's symptoms, which did not spread to other areas, fluctuated a little, but this seemed unrelated to any forms of treatment.

In fact, the few cases of obsessional neurosis in the elderly in which severe symptoms occur in the absence of depression have proved very intractable. In a recent case bifrontal leucotomy was narrowly avoided, when the patient's condition became tolerable after using a phenothiazine type drug in high dosage.

In concluding this chapter, it should be pointed out that character disorders, senile personality changes, psychosomatic and psycho-neurotic disorders have here been described in highly artificial isolation. Clinically, several of these disorders affect patients simultaneously, though usually one of them predominates. Cognitive deterioration sooner or later accompanies personality change; this and neurosis are often difficult to separate, and the intricate relation-ship between neurotic and affective disorders has been repeatedly stressed. The management of these persistent or frequently recurring conditions is palliative, and from occasion to occasion all available therapeutic measures are likely to find employment: psychotherapeutic support, psychiatric social work, periods of hospital care, domiciliary placement, occupational and social therapy, and even drug and physical treatments.

CHAPTER VII

MANAGEMENT
AND TREATMENT

METHODS of treatment were outlined in general terms in each of the chapters dealing with different clinical syndromes. A fuller discussion was postponed to avoid reduplications, arising from the fact that many currently used therapies are applicable to several disorders. In this last chapter an attempt will be made to present management and treatment in a systematic and comprehensive fashion. We suggest that the relationship established between patient and doctor at first contact, which is deepened during the diagnostic inquiry, should be discussed first and foremost. The severely ill patient is likely to be admitted to hospital, and psychiatric nursing will therefore be our next subject. Within or outside the hospital, occupational and social therapies are necessary adjuncts to psychiatric treatment. In the management of patients not requiring hospital admission, or of patients who have been discharged, psychiatric social work is of considerable importance. Having considered the different people concerned with the patient: the doctor, the nurse, the occupational therapist and the psychiatric social worker, we shall finally discuss the use of drugs and of forms of physical treatment. However, before attempting to deal with the treatment of established disorders, something must be said about prevention and prophylaxis.

PREVENTIVE TREATMENT

Unfortunately this section is going to be short; perhaps in future textbooks it will be longer. It is hardly necessary to point out that we know of no measures which will prevent or retard the progress of senile brain changes or of arterial degenerations—the main causes of so many mental disturbances seen in the elderly. Also, we have been at pains to show that emotional disorders such as depressions, paranoid states, personality changes and neuroses have their roots in earlier adult life or even in childhood. If it were possible to deal more effectively with the character disorders and emotional disturbances of younger people, if tendencies towards excessive introversion and emotional isolation could be reversed, if, in other words, the population could be rendered mentally healthier—then there might be a chance of reducing the heavy incidence of mental disturbances in later life which has been discovered in so many surveys.

While the actual prevention of psychological maladjustment and of mental illness in old age may be a Utopian dream, many prophylactic measures are available. Macmillan (1960) is convinced of this; he states, to give an example: "When the old person lives in isolation, either psychological (because of lack of interest, antagonism, self-pity or resentment on the part of relatives), or actual (because of solitude), deterioration sets in." Later on in the same paper he goes on: "When the emotional needs of the old person have been unsatisfied for any length of time, senile deterioration with subsequent onset of senile psychosis begins." In certain circumstances, Macmillan is even prepared to predict the time it takes, following emotional deprivation, for the psychosis to develop. One has seen too many old people become demented and affected by severe behaviour disorder, in spite of devoted and loving care from spouses and children, to accept such a simple theory of causation and prevention. However, many problems caused by senile dementia, and many social factors aggravating it, can be minimised by using the preventive methods advocated by Macmillan and other progressive psychiatrists and geriatricians. These apply mainly to the relatives of mentally deteriorating old people, whose attitude has been found to undergo a gradual change in many instances. At first responsibility is willingly accepted, but gradually the care of an old man or woman becomes increasingly irksome, especially when other relatives do not share the burden. Partial rejection results, and this tends to be converted into complete rejection by some special incidents, such as wandering away, nocturnal restlessness, incontinence, or accusatory talk and behaviour on the part of the old person. Once complete rejection has occurred, it is said to be irreversible, and when the patient has finally been admitted to hospital, relatives may often go to considerable lengths to avoid further responsibility. The remedy lies in discovering the occurrence of partial rejection, and of giving, at this early stage, relief to families by temporary admissions of the old person to hospital (especially for a holiday period). Other measures are attendance at a day hospital, or, in the case of less severely disorganised old people, at an occupational day centre. Furthermore, families should be allowed to feel that, when it comes to the worst, admission to hospital will be arranged. Macmillan claims that behaviour disorders like wandering away, accusatory and paranoid behaviour, nocturnal restlessness, and even certain types of urinary incontinence can in many cases be avoided by instituting this prophylactic regime. A necessary corollary is finding the early case. Within the framework of a community service, health visitors should pay especial attention to old people recently bereaved of their partners, as they are likely to develop reactions to emotional deprivation.

Many acute mental disturbances of the elderly are secondary to physical illnesses, and for this reason theoretically preventable. There is also reason to believe that gradual senile deterioration is speeded up by physical ill-health. Regular physical checkups, apart from making many medical emergencies less likely to occur, may also be of prophylactic value in the area of mental health.

Much publicity has been received by projects and courses intended to prepare people for old age, and there has also been a flood of inspirational publications. All these enterprises, including clubs and classes, no doubt help many people over potentially difficult years of readjustment, but it seems very doubtful whether they can prevent actual mental ill-health. The mentally and emotionally well-endowed person coming up against problems of retirement, financial limitations, bereavement, or ill-health, can fall back on inner resources, and will be able to seek and obtain support from people to whom he has related in a satisfactory and satisfying manner for many years. Persons with long-standing weaknesses of personality structure lack inner resilience, and have often failed to build up good relationships which will afford emotional support in times of crisis. These people are usually too insecure or too hostile to join in social activities or group projects, designed to promote new interests and satisfactions. In other words, people on the "danger list" for emotional disorders in late life are, on account of their make-up, unlikely to avail themselves of potentially preventive measures, however much these may be publicised. Whether modern methods of health education will be able to alter this unfortunate state of affairs remains to be seen.

THE FAMILY DOCTOR

We are once again thrown back on the necessity of discovering disturbances and deterioration at an early stage, and in this endeavour general practitioners should play the main role. The importance of recognising affective illnesses before they assume serious proportions and lead to suicidal acts has been heavily stressed in an earlier chapter. Lesser psychological disturbances are likely to give rise to complaints and nervous symptoms in the associates of elderly patients. Family doctors should not ignore these signs and are in the best possible position to discover the real causes of these disturbed family relationships. They may, at this early stage, be successful in getting the old person to take part in activities outside the home with a relief of tension, or the family doctor may be able to introduce a visitor to whom the patient can ventilate her grievances.

The general practitioner cannot possibly do any of these, and many other things, unless he is in frequent and regular contact with his elderly patients. They tend to consult their doctors much more frequently than younger people, and it is suggested that those who do not "bother" their doctors should be visited regularly. General practitioners who do this, and who maintain regular contacts with the family as well, claim that this type of care leads to a saving of doctors' time in the long run.

Patients expect three things from their doctors: (1) that he is interested in them and will give them sufficient time; (2) that he knows his job; (3) that he will remove their symptoms. All but the most disordered or the most unsophisticated elderly people will accept their doctor's lack of success in curing them, provided he remains interested in them and continues to give them his time and attention. Frank admission of failure on the doctor's part, as long as it is accompanied by proofs of continued interest, often turns out to be a useful therapeutic instrument, in that it places the patient in a position of superiority. As the doctor is usually younger than the patient, courteous deference on his part should come naturally and this will also enhance the patient's self esteem. Approached in this way, elderly patients who are often regarded as troublesome and demanding will often become grateful, appreciative and anxious not to make unnecessary and repetitive requests. These observations have led us to a consideration of the psychotherapeutic doctor–patient relationship.

PSYCHOTHERAPEUTIC MANAGEMENT

Raising the patient's self-esteem is one of the goals of a brief psychotherapeutic technique which Goldfarb (1956) has found useful in the management of argumentative, querulous, complaining, demanding and even suicide-threatening and aggressive old people, including those with evidence of brain damage. These disorders were often traced back to mounting helplessness, increasing feelings of worthlessness, and of anxiety. They could be understood as an accentuation of lifelong tendencies of looking upon other persons as on parent-surrogates, from whom to coax or command help. Sometimes it was possible for the therapist to assume the role of such a surrogate-parent who is permissive and non-punitive, as well as the provider of minor favours. However, most elderly patients were unable to increase their self-esteem and to decrease their sense of inferiority by developing the gratifying conviction of being loved by a parental figure. Their affectionate capacity appeared either poorly developed or had perhaps deteriorated. "With them it was essential to permit and encourage rapid development of an illusion that the therapist was a strong parental figure, that they were gaining him as a protective friend and ally, and that this was by the way of their own wit, wisdom, cunning, subtlety or other manifestation of personal strength. . . . The aim in each session with these persons was to have the patient leave with a conviction of "having" the therapist and of therefore taking along the protective powers of the omnipotent figure as well as a sense of triumph from his victory." Using this type of approach, Goldfarb achieved good success in one third of cases, was able to give support to a further third, but had to acknowledge failure in the remaining one third. Most patients responded to fewer than six sessions, lasting only 15 minutes each, and favourable results could be maintained by further widely spaced interviews (Goldfarb and Turner, 1953). Severe depressions, schizophrenic and paranoid illnesses did not benefit from this kind of management. According to a preliminary communication (Butler, 1960) the results of insight-orientated psychotherapy involving up to four or five sessions a week along psychoanalytic lines were also found disappointing in the case of elderly psychotics.

The doctor–patient relationship during more intensive psycho-therapy with elderly people (i.e. the transference situation) is discussed among others by Meerloo (1955), who gives a practical illustration:

> An elderly man developed an anxious–agitated illness following an operation, and was treated in 19 biweekly sessions using the technique of free association. During them the patient reported dreams concerning his childhood, as well as dreams which clearly portrayed preoccupations with death and un-willingness to die. (In one dream there occurred a number of manoeuvres to avoid catching a train due to depart on track 999.) Later on, when this patient was recovering, he dreamt of other people jumping out of the window, —i.e. he let other people go before him. In the transference situation, the author was the disciple, and the patient the teacher, who continued sending newspaper cuttings to the therapist long after the treatment was over.

Like other writers, Meerloo advises against any attempts at dissolving transferences with elderly patients, but suggests that some form of contact should be permitted indefinitely. Transference is easily built up with old people because they like the process of free association, which is closely related to senile talk. In it they regain control by going over childhood memories, and by seeing present events as determined by the past. The therapist best assumes the role of a benevolent super ego (or even of a pupil).

Referring to some seventy publications, Rechtschaffen (1959) in his review demonstrated that psychotherapeutic practice with the elderly had tended to develop away from orthodox psychoanalytic approaches, which were regarded as unsuited to subjects past the middle of life by Freud himself. Rechtschaffen traced this develop-ment into a continuum of aims which are far removed from the goals of intensive psychotherapy with younger people: (1) Insight approaches; (2) Supportive approaches; (3) Direct gratification and environmental modification; (4) Illusion-of-mastery therapy. He goes on to point out: "In general, the trend has been to use approaches toward the last named end of the continuum with the following characteristics of the aged being offered as reasons: the increased dependency which arises from realistically difficult circumstances;

the immodifiability of external circumstances to which a neurosis may be an optimal adjustive mechanism; irreversible impairment of intellectual and learning ability; resistance (or lack of resistance) to critical self-examination; the economics of therapeutic investment when life expectancy is shortened." Wayne (1952) has given some useful practical advice on how to conduct psychotherapy in senescence. In taking the history, special attention should be paid to understanding the patient's characteristic way of handling situations. On this background and on the assessment of the patient's mental status, the limited objectives of treatment should be tentatively formulated. Next, the focal current problem should be elicited (e.g. conflicts with children, resentment over retirement, etc.). Other problems usually surround the focal one, and they should be gradually drawn in the treatment. Some degree of insight might be aimed at, but basic character changes should not be expected, and old conflicts, especially in the sexual field, should not be rekindled. Wayne stresses that the therapist's approach must be genuinely warm and friendly. Pleasant personal remarks, which are taboo with younger patients, are definitely indicated. On the other hand, reactions of the patient to the therapist, like jealousy of other patients, patronising attitudes, plaintiveness and exaggerations of symptoms and attitudes, should all be pointed out (in contrast to what is recommended in Goldfarb's brief therapy). Wayne also suggests that it is useful to discuss the present position of the aged in society, as well as the process of ageing. Finally, treatment should be tailed off, but never officially concluded.

In the last chapter, we saw that disorders which are ordinarily regarded as particularly suitable for psychotherapy (the neuroses and personality problems) are relatively rarely seen in elderly people attending psychiatric clinics. However, it may well be that an approach to patients along psychotherapeutic lines, as just described, will enhance the efficacy of other therapeutic measures. The application of group therapy to geriatric hospital patients has been reported by several workers. Groups conducted by Silver (1950) and by Linden (from 1953 onwards, see Rechtschaffen's paper for summary of references) appear to have been meetings involving fairly large numbers of patients, and mainly didactic in character. Benaim (1957), working in our unit, reported on an open group run on non-directive lines, and attended at one time by from 7 to 10 patients. Most of them were recovering from depressive illnesses. Severely depressed patients voicing ideas of guilt or unworthiness were not acceptable to other group members, whereas people with circumscribed paranoid symptoms could be integrated. Topics in order of frequency discussed by the group were (1) the good old times; (2) social and economic difficulties; (3) feelings of rejection by one's own family; (4) complaints about the management of the ward and hospital; (5) the loneliness of old age; (6) physical complaints—by hypochondriacal patients only. By contrast, groups of younger psychoneurotic patients discussed subjects most frequently in the following order: (1) symptoms and anxieties; (2) sex; (3) marriage problems; (4) others in the group; (5) quarrels; (6) children (Talland and Clark, 1954). Some of the differences of topics which preoccupied young as against old patients are explained by the older patients suffering from more severe illnesses, but others are no doubt due to age differences. Sex discussions were positively rejected by the elderly group, and homosexuality was condemned unanimously, even though it had been a problem in a number of patients. In contrast to those of the younger neurotics, childhood memories tended to be happy. Group therapy in the elderly appears to have some value as a supportive measure. It is also a good way for the psychiatrist to find out more about his patients. For this reason, ward group meetings have become a weekly feature in our unit, and have been found to contribute towards a better therapeutic atmosphere.

NURSING

The chief agent in creating this therapeutic atmosphere is a well trained, and therefore insightful nursing staff. Most current psychiatric treatments can be given in consulting rooms and outpatient clinics. Hospital admission is obviously required in the case of physically ill or severely disabled patients. Otherwise, the main reason for recommending it lies in the realisation that the patient requires a therapeutically favourable milieu in addition to any specific psychological or somatic therapy. Suicidal tendencies apart, old people who live alone may have to be admitted. Also, many patients impose an unduly severe strain on their entourage because of agitated and importuning behaviour, or on account of the constant care and supervision required by many dements. In the earlier part of this chapter we discussed ways of dealing prophylactically with this situation, but in many instances continuous nursing care may eventually become necessary. Unless there are serious behaviour disorders, such as aggressive rages, episodes of noisy shouting, or severe restlessness, this should be given outside the mental hospital. A social stigma still attaches to psychiatric institutions and, more importantly, unnecessary admissions of senile persons with simple deterioration encroach upon the number of places for younger patients with more hopeful prognoses. There is everywhere a great need for more homes for the elderly confused, and for those with minor psychological aberrations, which make family care in modern living conditions so difficult or impossible. We shall not add to the flood of publications on this subject, as individual decisions on arranging care depend so much on the reader's local circumstances as well as on the patient's economic status. Unfortunately, conditions in these "last refuges", including some for well-to-do people, are often deplorable and much aggravated by unenlightened staff attitudes (Townsend, 1962).

A discussion of routine nursing techniques is outside the scope of this book, but we shall mention some ways in which doctors can help nurses and other attendants towards a better understanding of their work with deteriorated and disturbed old people. Much of the psychotic behaviour of the acutely confused at any age is due to severe fear generated by disorientation, misidentification of people, and misapprehensions about the situation; the presence of frightening hallucinations is a much less important factor in most cases. In allaying these states of panic, which through exhaustion are the main causes of death, good nursing is the most important factor. Pending the removal by medical or surgical means of any underlying physical causes of the delirium, good nursing acts much more efficiently than drugs with their undesirable side- and after-effects. Alexander Kennedy (1959) has stressed the importance of restoring some degree of orientation to patients in senile delirium. He describes how they wake fitfully after the first exhausted sleep "in an unrecognised world of threatening shadows and sounds of evil portent. The observer soon discovers that he must repeatedly say who he is, explain the surroundings to his patient with a minimum of words and comment on any noises or movements that catch his fleeting attention. If he does this and follows the muttered and whispered words which reveal what the patient is thinking about, he will find that, as a recognised and friendly presence, he provides a focal point about which the patient can orientate his thoughts. Relief of fear and with it sleep may come from his quiet reassurance." In the nursing of delirious patients the following points should be borne in mind: the environment should be stabilised by keeping the bed in the same place and by providing visible furniture features. According to Kennedy, orientation is improved by strong multicoloured decorations and by importing familiar possessions. Changes of staff should be minimal. Introductions of people should be repeated, shadows avoided. Talk and explanations should be repetitive and in a quiet reassuring tone of voice. Visits from the family should be brief, and discussion should be limited to matters of the well-remembered past. This sort of approach may be impracticable in severely delirious patients, but even they are likely to pass through more lucid episodes, during which a nurse who is constantly with the patient will have opportunities of making reassuring and orientating contacts.

The nursing of elderly patients with affective and schizophrenic illnesses differs hardly from that of younger psychotics. The motherly attitudes which many nurses almost instinctively adopt towards aged people may serve well with some. In others, a deferential attitude allowing the patient to believe that he or she is the master of the situation may be found more appropriate. Regular conferences of psychiatrists with the nursing staff, in which all new patients are discussed, and in which all arising problems can be ventilated, have been found indispensable. Some elderly patients can be very trying, and punitive nursing attitudes tend to create even more disturbed and histrionic behaviour. These undesirable staff reactions are less likely to occur when nurses know more about their patients and the deeper causes of their behaviour.

Demented patients require careful observation of their physical state and much general nursing. Regular encouragement to the toilet may avoid loss of sphincter control, or partially restore it. Constant stimulation towards activity, in between adequate rest periods, is essential. This will be discussed in the next section. The great majority of deteriorating old people are quite rightly looked after in various homes and institutions, which rarely employ nurses with psychiatric training. The attitudes of these untrained or partially trained staffs need careful watching, and doctors who arrange long term care for elderly people should familiarise themselves with the various homes in their area and with the people running them; tolerance of aberrant behaviour varies greatly from person to person. Townsend (1962) found many matrons to be rather unimaginative and authoritarian, even though they were well disposed towards their charges and took good physical care of them. Doctors familiar with the problems of old people should be asked to take part in the training and supervision of the staffs for homes for the aged. One finds in these staffs one or the other of two opposing attitudes, which are equally unhelpful (Goldfarb, 1953): the one is excessively hostile and belittling, i.e. the feeling that old people are slovenly, deteriorated, hopeless and even repulsive cases; the other, too compassionate and too loving. It is suggested that these attitudes arise from anxieties caused, either by a feeling that old people make too many demands on us and present problems which make us feel helpless and perhaps angry, or by reminders of what may happen to us, of our own vulnerability and mortality; this makes us irrationally and excessively compassionate. It is suggested that these unhelpful attitudes can be altered by giving nurses and attendants a better understanding of the causes of aberrant behaviour—of the frustrations and deprivations, and of the increased dependency or resentment of some elderly people. Abnormal behaviour will not then be regarded as a personal threat, arousing anxiety and irrational attitudes, but in each case as a challenge to discover its causes. Staffs will thus be encouraged to diminish their charges' sense of deprivation, helplessness, need of excessive dependency, or whatever else is discovered, by putting into use the old person's residual assets. This brings us to our next subject:

OCCUPATIONAL AND RE-SOCIALISING THERAPIES

In the treatment of recoverable psychiatric illnesses, occupational therapy is a useful aid. The beneficial effects of a period away from family stresses, of psychotherapeutic support, and of somatic therapies might easily be counterbalanced by boredom and self-absorption. Well-run psychiatric units have daily programmes of ward chores, social activities and handicraft sessions, in which all patients take part under the joint guidance of occupational therapists and nurses. With younger patients, who are likely to return to a job and who may well require occupational resettlement in a new skill, therapy should be as realistic and utilitarian as possible in hospital surroundings. Old patients may often require guidance in the opposite direction, towards "disengagement" from work by taking up substitute activities. Many of these patients may carry on with craft-work like rugmaking or basketry, which they learnt during a psychiatric illness, in their own homes or in clubs for ex-patients. Sheltered workshops and occupational day centres, which produce an output of paid light industrial work (e.g. simple assembly jobs), may be more acceptable to bored and lonely elderly persons without actual psychiatric disorders. Whichever the setting, work should be relieved by play, and once a working group has been formed, other socialising activities are easily introduced. Unfortunately, persons prone to develop psychological disorders experience great difficulties in joining clubs or in bringing themselves to attend day centres, even when there are adequate transport facilities. Energetic and persistent social workers are needed to persuade and guide elderly people of this type towards these activities.

In the treatment of senile dements, the value of organised ward programmes with occupational, recreational and work therapy has been investigated by several groups of workers. The introduction of these methods in an American state hospital led to a 300 per cent increase of the discharge rate (Rechtschaffen *et al.*, 1953). Follow-up of patients demonstrated, however, that there had been no improvement on a behaviour rating scale. The increased discharge rate had probably been the result of increased efforts of placing patients out of hospital, which had been concomitant with the introduction of an intensive treatment programme (Atkinson *et al.*, 1955). In working with elderly dements, institutionally cared for outside the mental hospital, we were able to demonstrate that "pushing" different types of social and simple occupational therapy led on each occasion to an improvement of behaviour ratings. Scores dropped again as soon as patients were left to their own devices though the activities were still visibly available to them. Comparing subjects with a control group, there was no significant change for the better after treatments had continued over from nine to twelve months. We concluded that demented patients, in addition to other and more obvious defects, also lacked self motivation. If made to occupy themselves, they can be maintained at a higher level, and will present a less distressing picture to their visiting friends (Cosin *et al.*, 1958). Quite apart from

6

the palliative role of occupational and social therapy in persistently confused old people, its introduction will increase the morale of the nursing staff. Simple domestic tasks and craft work, together with group activities like sing-songs, collection of newspaper items and outings, were found to be equally acceptable. All of these activities are easily initiated and supervised by nurses, with little professional guidance from occupational therapists.

Many mentally deteriorating old people suffer from locomotor disabilities and are psychologically helped by physiotherapy; even speech therapy may be useful in certain cases of dysphasia due to cerebral arteriosclerosis (Mitchell, 1958).

PSYCHIATRIC SOCIAL WORK

Increased deployment of social workers, within a framework of improved community care of the elderly, would no doubt avoid or delay removal of old people from their own homes (Townsend, 1962). Extension of social work was advocated by Macmillan (1960) as a means of instituting early treatment of senile deterioration and of avoiding rejection of old persons by their families. The great after-care needs of elderly psychiatric patients, many of whom make only partial recoveries or have recurring disturbances, have been highlighted recently (Freeman and Farndale, 1963).

The Psychiatric Social Worker has two additional tasks, which superficially may appear to differ, but which in reality are closely interrelated: (1) Social assessment and practical arrangements; (2) Dealing with problems between the patient and his family. Psychiatric patients may need help with financial matters, as they may be unable to claim the appropriate pension or assistance on account of their illness. Attitudes of other people at work or in the neighbourhood may require investigation. However, the main task of the P.S.W. in this area will be the patient's correct placement on discharge from hospital, or in order to avoid psychiatric admission. With many elderly psychiatric patients recovery is incomplete, but relapses may be prevented by placing them in a suitable environment, especially when they had been living alone or with relatives unwilling or unable to cope with residual symptoms. Much work is entailed in finding suitable homes and institutions, and in arranging the patient's acceptance. This is not just a routine task, because the world of the mentally impaired old person has often shrunk to their room and to the people with whom they have been in daily contact. Much persuasion may be needed before an alternative is accepted, and many elderly patients will refuse to leave their homes and will insist on returning to quite unsuitable surroundings. In these circumstances the P.S.W. will have to visit the patient following discharge, in order to keep an eye on the situation.

The other sphere of the P.S.W.'s activities lies in therapeutic work with the patient's family. At younger ages, psychiatric disturbances are often found to be connected with psychological disorders in other members of a patient's social orbit, and it may sometimes be difficult to decide whether the patient who is referred for treatment is in fact the sickest person in a family group. In a recent study, younger people with neurotic personalities and chronic or frequently recurring affective reactions were found to have associated significantly more often with other psychologically disturbed persons than was the case in acute psychotics with previously stable personalities. Offspring were more likely to be psychiatrically abnormal than spouses or other members of the patient's entourage (Post, 1962a).

It is not therefore surprising that elderly people with depressive reactions of a long-standing and neurotic type, are often found living with other persons, especially their children, who on closer acquaintance turn out to have psychological problems of their own. In fact, one may discover reverberating circuits of psychopathological interaction, and work of the Psychiatric Social Workers with members of the patient's family may be urgently indicated.

The P.S.W.'s therapeutic contribution was recently investigated in a sample of female patients over 60 (Colwell and Post, 1963). Almost all were suffering from affective and neurotic disorders and the great majority had shown milder personality disorders throughout life. Many were widows, and case-work was concerned mainly with one of their children. As one might expect, daughters were most frequently affected. Therapeutic technique varied from case to case, but dealing with practical matters often proved a useful way of opening up the situation. Interviews were conducted as a rule with the patient, and with her daughter or son separately; but of greatest interest, on account of the insights they permitted, were sessions in which the patient, her daughter, the psychiatrist and the P.S.W. took part. These meetings were found to be therapeutic when they enabled the patient and her daughter to ventilate their negative feelings for one another, which each had expressed so clearly to their doctor and to the P.S.W. With both therapists present, it was possible to explain the interaction in a guilt-reducing fashion, and realistic arrangements for the future were made acceptable. In many instances, a number of lengthy interviews had to be conducted with the patient, the daughter, and with both together following the patient's discharge from hospital. In these sessions much of the stormy past was relived and related to the present and to the future.

It could be demonstrated that the psychopathology of mothers and their offspring was often complementary. Patients thought that children ran their lives badly and disapproved of their choice of marriage partners. They often felt that their children made too many demands on them, did not give enough in return, and expected too much gratitude. Envy of the children's greater intelligence and higher educational as well as social status was often ill-concealed. Children on the other hand, were often ashamed of their parents. They also found that they made too many demands on them, and that they were too possessive. In fact, daughters were frequently over-dependent, married late or not at all. One even dared not have a child, for fear of what her mother would say. Hostility and guilt were marked components of the daughters' feelings for their mothers.

Really good results were obtained in only nine of the 32 cases in this sample. With others, some improvements were produced, mainly in the direction of promoting agreed detachment of parent from child (e.g. with the parent moving into a suitable home). Complete failure was experienced in eight cases; in practically all of them, the daughter or son were regarded by the psychiatrist as suffering from definite psychiatric illnesses. Low intelligence, and perhaps also low social class, were other factors militating against success in this form of family therapy.

SOMATIC THERAPIES

The presence of physical ill-health affects prognosis of any psychiatric illness adversely, but we cannot here discuss the treatment of physical disorders in elderly psychiatric patients. We shall have to limit ourselves to considering somatic therapies which are thought to affect cerebral functioning through (1) medicinal substances;

(2) artificial epileptiform discharges (electroconvulsive therapy); and (3) surgical interruption of intracerebral connections (psychosurgery).

Full discussion of all somatic therapies advocated during the last decade would fill a separate volume, and would bewilder the reader without helping him in the treatment of his patients. Therefore, I shall present only those methods which I have found useful, and which I believe to have largely contributed towards changing geriatric psychiatry into a branch of clinical medicine in which worthwhile therapeutic results can be obtained. However, somatic therapies have been left for discussion to the end of this chapter, because they act most effectively in a setting of a good relationship of the patient with the doctor and his auxiliary workers. Furthermore, much evidence has accumulated (Weatherall, 1962) demonstrating that therapies are significantly more effective when doctors believe in their efficacy.

In this section, I shall be making a series of brief, personal and I fear rather dogmatic statements, and shall probably omit some methods of treatment which may have given excellent result in other hands. On account of the rapidly changing climate of opinion concerning the value of drugs in psychiatry, only few references to the literature will be quoted. Pursuing this dogmatic approach, a few general rules are here recommended:

(1) Employ only a few methods of treatment, and do not try out everything as soon as reports begin to appear. In this way you will become intimately acquainted with each therapy, and especially with each drug and its undesirable side effects.

(2) With each individual patient, draw up an explicit plan of treatment, and follow it through. Your mistakes may then appear clearly, and you may learn to avoid them in future.

(3) Dosage and time during which any therapy may be expected to act should be known to you; do not, therefore, change over to a different form of treatment, too soon.

(4) On the other hand, do not allow "therapeutic perseveration" to occur. In the event of therapeutic failure, review all the evidence, and be prepared to change your original plan of campaign.

(5) Except as a last resort, do not use several allegedly specific therapies at the same time. In employing a blunderbuss approach you may be lucky and obtain quick results. However, the patient will be the loser in the long run; in our age group, most of them will have

6*

further attacks, and it will be helpful to know which form of treatment has helped in the past, and is likely to be effective in the future.

With the exception of replacement therapies in psychoses due to deficiency states, and of antibiotic treatments of infections of the central nervous systems causing mental symptoms (first and foremost G.P.I.), all current somatic treatments in psychiatry probably act only symptomatically. They abolish or diminish disorders of mood, experiencing and thinking, as well as behaviour disorders associated with them. We do not treat illnesses, but only symptoms.

Sleep disturbances in elderly people, except those suffering from delirious reactions and from severe functional psychoses, usually respond to one of the following preparations: Chloral hydrate can now be administered in tablet or acceptable liquid form as a compound with phenazone: dichloralphenazone ("Welldorm"). The normal hypnotic dose is two 10-grain tablets, but this may be increased to four. An alternative preparation is cycloheptonyl barbituric acid ("Medomin") 200–400 mg. The change may be rung with amylobarbitone sodium ("Sodium Amytal") in a dosage of 100–300 mg. A more powerful combination consists of quinalbarbitone sodium 100 mg, with amylobarbitone sodium 100 mg ("Tuinal"); in cases of severe sleeplessness, a double dose may prove effective. There are many other preparations, but these have been found to produce more drowsiness next morning.

When *acute confusional states* are not caused by toxic or anoxic factors, they are sometimes due to specific deficiencies. Replacement therapies employed in myxoedema, alcoholic psychoses, subacute combined degeneration, etc. do not differ from those used in younger patients. In the treatment of non-specific senile delirious reactions, massive dosage with vitamins is usually advocated, even when patients do not exhibit signs of specific vitamin deficiencies. In the latter case, the efficacy of this treatment is difficult to prove, but in the present state of knowledge, a short and intensive course of potent mixtures of vitamins intravenously or intramuscularly administered, should not be withheld. The manufacturers' instructions should be followed. Some workers continue to try to improve cerebral metabolism by intravenous infusions of 10 per cent glucose in normal saline, 1–2 litres at a rate of 50 drops per minute, daily.

The paramount importance of good and psychologically orientated nursing was stressed earlier in this chapter, but some chemical form of sedation is required as well. Slowly acting and slowly excreted substances, such as most barbiturates and bromides, must be avoided as they will literally make "confusion worse confounded". Paraldehyde used to be the best drug available, preferably administered by mouth (4–8 ml.), or by injection deeply into the vastus lateralis of the thigh (Injectio Paralhydi, 5–10 ml.). Methyl-pentynol ("Oblivon") up to 1·5 grammes had a recent vogue for the less severe types of sleeplessness in senile confusional states.

The modern treatment of *behaviour disorders in acute and chronic brain syndromes* is with one of the so-called tranquillising drugs. In their use, sudden hypotensive effects must be watched for. Jaundice, permanent liver damage, and aplastic anaemias were greater problems with the earlier preparations, but these complications must still be kept in mind. Parkinsonian symptoms will frequently appear, but unless the dosage has been excessively high, they are well controlled by the appropriate drugs, and reversible. It is generally thought that promazine hydrochloride ("Sparine") is the safest preparation for senile persons. It may be given intramuscularly or intravenously in an initial dose of 50 mg, which may be repeated after ten minutes. In severely disturbed patients, up to 400 mg daily may be given in this way, but with this high dosage Llewellyn (1961) found a vicious cycle of restlessness–sleep–drowsiness–restlessness established, which favoured the occurrence of urinary incontinence, bedsores and contractures. He recommended maintenance therapy with promazine resinate ("Sparine Latab") 50 mg twice daily; if necessary, this dosage may be increased to 500 mg a day. Phenothiazine drugs have, as one might expect, not been found useful in patients with apathy, incontinence and confusion due to chronic brain syndromes (Hamilton and Bennett, 1962). Restless behaviour only is controlled by these preparations, when used for the treatment of organic psychosyndromes.

Many tranquillisers have found application in the treatment of *manic states*. A substituted butyrophenone, haliperidol ("Serenace") has been found suitable for controlling symptoms in most cases, without troublesome side effects. In an emergency it may be given intramuscularly or intravenously in a dosage of 5 mg and repeated 6-hourly. Adequate control of geriatric manic patients can usually be maintained on 1·5–3·0 mg daily.

Schizophrenic-paranoid symptoms in the elderly almost always respond to phenothiazine drugs. Trifluoperazine ("Stelazine") should be started with a dosage of 5 mg twice daily; after a week or two this may have to be increased by 5 mg steps, every two to three weeks, until hallucinatory experiences disappear and delusional ideas are no longer expressed. At this stage the daily dose can usually be reduced, and it may finally be possible to stabilise the patient on a daily intake of 3–5 mg; this can be taken in a single dose. Long term supervision and readjustment of dosage are esssential, and we have found that in an occasional patient treatment can be ultimately discontinued (for a preliminary account, see Post, 1962b). Unfortunately, trifluoperazine has several unpleasant side effects, which in my experience cannot always be avoided or abolished by adjusting dosage. Parkinsonian symptoms are easily controlled, but unpleasant sensations of restlessness and visible hyperkinetic disorders (akathesia) can remain very troublesome; some patients also complain of depression, anergia and apathy to a disabling extent. On preliminary impression, these side effects may be avoided by using thioridazine ("Melleril"), commencing with 50 mg three times daily, and increasing gradually up to 600 mg daily. There are risks of retinal damage with a prolonged daily dosage exceeding 800–1000 mg but no evidence of fundal changes or of visual impairment was found in over 100 patients treated with Melleril for up to five years within the recommended dosage range of 150–600 mg daily (Remy, 1962). It has to be admitted that an occasional elderly paranoid patient has failed to improve significantly on these and other phenothiazine preparations on account of serious side or toxic effect with each of them. As was discussed earlier (Chapter VI) the borders between schizophrenia and melancholia are often indistinct, and the use of antidepressive measures alongside with phenothiazines may have to be seriously considered.

Though many *depressive states* will recover or improve without any specific somatic therapy, it is not now usual to assume an expectant attitude of masterly inactivity; depression entails considerable suffering and, suicidal risks apart, patients are prone to develop serious secondary physical illnesses while they are in a depressed state. Electroconvulsive therapy can be expected to produce early remission of symptoms in some 80 per cent of elderly depressives. The convulsions are now usually modified by muscle relaxants, and old age, provided there have not been recent cardiac infarcts or serious cardio-respiratory failure, is no contraindication to this form of treatment. There is no advantage in administering electro-convulsive treatments more frequently than twice a week, and they should be spaced out further as soon as there are signs of a remission. It is probably pointless to give more than 12–14 treatments in one consecutive set. Memory impairment usually occurs, but almost always recovers after a few weeks.

Claims of success with any of the so-called antidepressive drugs have hardly ever exceeded a rate of 65 per cent. They do not appear to produce a genuine remission of the illness (as is sometimes claimed for ECT), but only a very considerable improvement of anxious and depressive affect and thought content. Eventually, the depressive illness runs its course to a natural end, and the drug can then be discontinued. Sometimes the patients know when this point has been reached, but in most cases it is necessary to observe the effects of lowering their dosage. In this age group, patients may go on for several years having recurrences of symptoms as soon as treatment is discontinued. Personally, I have found imipramine hydrochloride ("Tofranil") the most useful preparation in this group. Starting with 25 mg three times a day, the dose can in a few days be raised to 50, and later even to 75 mg thrice daily. Therapeutic effects are not seen during the first week or ten days; they may be delayed for three or four weeks. Many patients experience side effects, such as dryness of mouth, sweating and tremulousness. As with other antidepressive drugs, a very occasional patient develops a blood dyscrasia or liver damage. In elderly people, mild delirious states with a visual hallucinosis have been very occasionally encountered. The less serious of these complications do not contraindicate continuation of treatment at a lower dosage. Of the monoamine oxidase inhibitors, tranylcypromine sulphate ("Parnate"), or 10 mg of this substance in combination with 1 mg of trifluoperazine ("Parstelin") have been found therapeutically active in anxious-depressive patients. Dosage is 10 mg twice a day, and it is not safe to exceed this. Improvement should become apparent after a few days, and there is no point in continuing this preparation in the absence of beneficial effects after more than two weeks. The occurrence of headaches should be a signal for discontinuing it; a high intake of protein, especially cheese, should be avoided.

In mildly depressed patients, or in those who can be adequately supervised at home, a trial of one or even two drugs is an obvious first choice, especially as most patients are apprehensive of electroconvulsive therapy. When hospital admission has been necessary for clinical or social reasons, a decision will have to be reached whether the patient is more likely to respond to ECT or to drug treatment. A preliminary investigation, in which elderly depressives were randomised for treatment with either ECT or imipramine, showed that ECT produced a higher immediate remission rate, but during the subsequent three months a number of patients relapsed. Late results with the drug were a little better, but this might have been due to an increasing number of remissions occurring during an observation period of four months. By and large, ECT and imipramine were equally effective in a high proportion of cases, and in some both failed. Analysis of our findings has not so far brought to light any aspects of the clinical picture or previous personality of elderly depressives which correlated with better results with either imipramine or electroconvulsive therapy. As the last of these produces early improvement with greater certainty, we tend to employ it as a first choice in acutely and severely depressed patients, while reserving drug therapy for those who relapse. We tend to use drugs as an initial treatment for patients who are only moderately ill.

Psychosurgery retains a very definite place in the treatment of the persistent depressions of old age. Freeman (1962) reminded us that among the first cases reported by the originators of lobotomy there were several patients over the age of 60. Thorpe (1958) reviewed the results obtained with Freeman and Watt's standard prefrontal leucotomies in 50 consecutive patients over 65. Even with this early type of operation, there were only one postoperative death and four cases with cerebral sequelae (fits, serious in two). Of the 49 surviving patients, 35 made full and lasting affective remissions and only one paranoid patient showed no improvement. Twenty-one of 32 patients surviving for more than five years remained completely well. Thorpe (1960) and Freeman (1962) claim even better results with more recent, restricted surgical techniques. Probably, a proportion of the patients reported by these workers had not been ill for very long, and had been leucotomised because ECT had been thought contraindicated for physical reasons. Our practice has been to reserve the operation for patients who had been continuously ill, without any remissions, for at least 18 months, and who had had several courses of electroconvulsive treatment. They had remained tense, depressed and agitated, without signs of cerebral disease, and long term mental hospital care seemed likely to be required. Patients with aggressive and acting-out tendencies in their premorbid personalities, and those with unsatisfactory social backgrounds tended to be excluded. For all these reasons, relatively few patients have come to operation (open bimedial leucotomy), and only 16 have so far been followed over three years. Ten have made complete and lasting recoveries, but four had to be classed as complete failures. Two patients became incapacitated by postoperative cerebral complications, and three patients showed troublesome personality changes. Mild frontal lobe syndromes were not infrequently encountered, but lasted for only a few months. The present position may be summarised as follows: even using modern techniques, leucotomy is attended by very definite risks; but these can be accepted, provided the operation is reserved as a last resort in apparently incurable agitated depressions. No opinion can as yet be offered concerning the value of leucotomy in elderly people with frequently recurring depressive and manic attacks.

CLOSING REMARKS

We have seen that there are many ways in which elderly people with psychological disturbances can be helped, and that in most of them three sets of causal factors can be discerned: (1) Lifelong personality developments within a network of relationships with others; (2) senescent changes, especially those affecting the brain; and (3) disorders of mood, thinking, experiencing and behaving, probably arising from constitutional predispositions.

My aim has been to demonstrate that it is both necessary and possible to determine for each patient which of these sets of factors contributes most strongly in producing a psychological disorder. Only in this way will it be possible to formulate a plan of action, which will contain one chief therapeutic aim and several subsidiary ones. When psychological problems arise mainly from character changes and conflicts with other persons in the family, our approach will be largely psychotherapeutic, but we shall also employ other means to improve the patient's relationships, and may have to deal with any affective or paranoid disturbances present. Our method of approach will depend on the patient's level of intellectual preservation. In the case of dementing patients, control of affective or schizophreniform symptoms may also be necessary, but our main efforts will be towards mobilising the patient's remaining assets. Arrangements for his future care will very much depend on the state of the patient's interpersonal relationships. Finally, affective or schizophrenic states will be treated *secundum artem*, but much more successfully if we are able to establish a good relationship with the patient, and if we can improve the quality of his contacts with other people. The type and intensity of specific therapies will depend on his general physical and cerebral states.

Sometimes, we may effect cures; frequently, we may be able to ameliorate the patient's condition; we shall always endeavour to give him and his family sympathetic support. In epigrammatic form:

Quelquefois guérir; soulager souvent; consoler toujours.

REFERENCES

ABRAHAM, G. (1962) Pensée et peur de la mort chez les vieillards atteints de troubles mentaux, *Schweiz. Arch. Neurol. Neurochirurg. & Psychiat.*, **90**, 362.

ALBERT, ELFRIEDE (1960) Das Altern, insbesondere die Hirnalterung als zellulaeres Problem und seine biochemischen Aspekte, *Fortschr. Neurol. Psychiat.*, **28**, 423.

ALBRECHT, RUTH (1951) Social roles in the prevention of senility, *J. Gerontol.*, **6**, 380.

ALLISON, R. S. (1962) *The Senile Brain: A Clinical Study*, Edward Arnold, London.

ARNHOFF, F. N. (1961) Concepts of Ageing in *Psychopathology of Ageing*, Hoch, P.H. and Zubin, J. (eds.) Grune & Stratton, New York.

ATKINSON, S., FJELD, S. P., and FREEMAN, J. G. (1953) The intensive treatment program for state hospital geriatric patients. II. Further progress and results, *Geriatrics*, **10**, 111.

AVERY, L. W. (1945) Common factors precipitating mental symptoms in the aged, *Arch. Neurol. Psychiat.*, **54**, 312.

BARTLETT, J. E. A. (1951) Hallucinations in an old man with cataracts, *Brain*, **74**, 363.

BENAIM, S. (1956) *A Clinical Study of Obsessional Illnesses in Old Age*. Dissertation for the Academic Postgraduate Diploma in Psychological Medicine of the University of London.

BENAIM, S. (1957) Group therapy within a geriatric unit: An experiment, *Internat. J. Soc. Psychiat.*, **3**, 123.

BENDER, L. (1938) *A Visual-Motor Gestalt Test and its Clinical Use*, Research Monograph No. 3, Amer. Orthopsychiat. Ass., New York.

BERNER, P. and HOFF, H. (1959) Krisen des Altwerdens, *Vita Hum.*, **2**, 166.

BIRREN, J. E. (1960) Behavioral theories of ageing, in *Ageing*, Amer. Ass. for the Advancement of Science.

BIRREN, J. E. (1961) Research in the psychology of ageing: concepts and findings, in *Psychopathology of Ageing*, Hoch, P. H. and Zubin, J. (eds.), Grune & Stratton, New York.

BLEULER, M. (1943) Die Spaetschizophrenen Krankheitsbilder, *Fortschr. Neurol. & Psychiat.*, **15**, 259.

BLEULER, M. (1954) Psychiatry of cerebral diseases, *Brit. Med. J.*, **2**, 1233.

BONDAREFF, W. (1959) Morphology of the ageing nervous system, in BIRREN, J. E., *Handbook of Ageing and the Individual*, University of Chicago Press.

BOTWINNICK, J. and BIRREN, J. (1951) Differential decline in the Wechsler–Bellevue sub-tests in the senile psychoses, *J. Gerontol.*, **6**, 365.

BRIERLEY, J. B. (1961) Clinico-pathological correlations in amnesia, *Geront. Clin.*, **3**, 97.

BROWN, C. C., GANTT, W. M. and WHITMAN, J. R. (1961) Measures of adaptability in senility, in *Psychopathology of Ageing*, Hoch, P. H. and Zubin, J. (eds.), Grune & Stratton, New York.

BUERGER, M. (1958) Der Desoxyribonucleinsaeure-und Ribonucleinsaeuregehalt des menschlichen Gehirns im Laufe des Lebens, *Z. Altersforsch.*, **12**, 123.

BURNET, M. (1959) Auto-immune disease, *Brit. Med. J.*, **2**, 645.

BUSSE, E. W. (1961) Psychoneurotic reactions and defense mechanisms in the aged, in *Psychopathology of Ageing*, Hoch, P. H., and Zubin, J. (eds.), Grune & Stratton, New York.

BUSSE, E. W., BARNES, R. H., SILVERMAN, H. J., THALER, M. and FROST, L. L. (1955) Studies of the process of ageing, X. The strength and weaknesses of psychic functioning in the aged, *Amer. J. Psychiat.*, **111**, 896.

BUSSE, E. W., DOVENMUEHLE, R. D., and BROWN, R. G. (1960) Psychoneurotic reactions of the aged, *Geriatrics*, **15**, 97.

BUTLER, R. N. (1960) Intensive psychotherapy for the hospitalised aged, *Geriatrics*, **15**, 644.

CAIRD, W. K. and INGLIS, J. (1961) The short-term storage of auditory and visual two-channel digits by elderly patients with memory disorder, *J. Ment. Sci.*, **107**, 1062.

CAMERON, D. E. (1941) Studies in senile nocturnal delirium, *Psychiat. Quart.*, **15**, 47.

CAMERON, D. E. (1958) The use of nucleic acid in aged patients with memory impairment, *Amer. J. Psychiat.*, **114**, 943.

CAMERON, D. E. and SOLYOM, G. (1961) Effects of ribonucleic acid on memory, *Geriatrics*, **16**, 74.

CAMERON, D. E., SOLYOM, G., SVED, S. and WAINRIB, B. (1962) Effects of intravenous administration of ribonucleic acid upon failure of memory for recent events in presenile and aged individuals. Unpublished paper.

CAMERON, N. (1956) The Neuroses of Later Maturity, in *Mental Disorders in Late Life*, Kaplan, O. J. (ed.), Stanford University Press.

COLWELL, CATHERINE, and POST, F. (1959) Community needs of elderly psychiatric patients, *Brit. Med. J.*, **2**, 214.

COLWELL, CATHERINE, and POST, F. (1963) The parent–child relationship in the treatment of elderly psychiatric patients. Paper read to the *Sixth International Congress of Gerontology*, Copenhagen.

COMFORT, A. (1961) The position of fundamental age studies, *Amer. Heart J.*, **62**, 293.

CORSELLIS, J. A. N. (1962) *Mental Illness and the ageing Brain*, Maudsley Monograph No. 9, Oxford University Press, London.

CORSELLIS, J. A. N. and EVANS, P. E. (1963) Observations on the relation of vascular disease to cerebral degeneration and to mental disorders in old age. Paper read to the *Social Research Seminar, Sixth International Congress of Gerontology* (to be published).

COSIN, L. Z., MORT, MARGARET, POST, F., WESTROPP, CELIA, and WILLIAMS, MOYRA (1958) Experimental treatment of persistent senile confusion, *Internat. J. Soc.* Psychiat., **4**, 24.

CUMMING, ELAINE, and HENRY, W. E. (1961) *Growing Old*, Basic Books Inc., New York.

DIETHELM, O. and ROCKWELL, F. V. (1943) Psychopathology of ageing, *Amer. J. Psychiat.*, **99**, 553.

DINGMAN, W. and SPORN, M. B. (1961) The incorporation of 8-azaguanine into rat brain RNA and its effect on maze-learning by the rat; An inquiry into the biochemical basis of memory, *J. Psychiat. Res.*, **1**, 1.

DORKEN, H. (1958) Normal senescent decline and senile dementia: Their differentiation by psychological test, *Med. Serv. J. Canada*, **14**, 18.

DOUST, J. W., SCHNEIDER, R. A., TALLAND, G. A., WALSH, M. A., and BARKER, G. B. (1953) The correlation between intelligence and anoxaemia in senile dementia, *J. nerv. Ment. Dis.*, **117**, 383.

EAST, N. W. (1944) Crime, senescence and senility, *J. Ment. Sci.*, **90**, 835.

EXTON-SMITH, A. N. (1961) Terminal illness in the aged, *Lancet*, **2**, 305.

FISH, F. (1960) Senile schizophrenia, *J. Ment. Sci.*, **106**, 938.

FISHER, M. (1951) Occlusion of the internal carotid artery, *A.M.A. Arch. Neurol. & Psychiat.*, **65**, 346.

FISHER, M. (1954) Occlusion of the carotid arteries: Further experiences, *A.M.A. Arch. Neurol. & Psychiat.*, **72**, 187.

FREEMAN, H. and FARNDALE, J. (eds.) (1963) *Trends in the Mental Health Services*, Pergamon Press, Oxford.

FREEMAN, W. (1962) Lobotomy after 65, *Geriatrics*, **17**, 15.

FREY, T. S. and SJOEGREN, H. (1959) The electroencephalogram in elderly persons suffering from neuropsychiatric disorders, *Act. Psychiat. Neurol. Scand.*, **34**, 438.

FULLER, G. B. and LAIRD, J. T. (1963) The Minnesota Percepto-diagnostic test, *J. Clin. Psychol.*, **19**, 3, Sp. Mono. Supp. 16.

GASSTER, M. (1961) Clinical experience with L-Glutavite in aged patients with behaviour problems and memory defects, *J. Amer. Geriat. Soc.*, **9**, 370.

GILBERT, J. G. (1941) Memory loss in senescence, *J. abnorm. soc. Psychol.*, **36**, 73.

GINZBERG, R. (1955) Sleep and sleep disturbances in geriatric psychiatry, *J. Amer. Geriat. Soc.*, **3**, 493.

GOLDFARB, A. I. (1953) The orientation of staff in a home for the aged, *Ment. Hygiene*, **37**, 76.

GOLDFARB, A. I. (1956) Psychotherapy of the aged, *Psychoanalyt. Rev.*, **43**, 68.

GOLDFARB, A. I. and TURNER, HELEN (1953) Psychotherapy of aged persons: II. Utilization and effectiveness of "brief" therapy, *Amer. J. Psychiat.*, **109**, 916.

GOLDSTEIN, K. (1939) *The Organism*, Am. Book Co., New York.

GOSLING, R. H. (1955) The association of dementia with radiologically demonstrated cerebral atrophy, *J. Neurol. Neurosurg. Psychiat.*, **18**, 129.

GRAHAM, F. K. and KENDALL, BARBARA S. (1960) Memory-for-designs Test: revised general manual. *Percept. Mot. Skills*, **11**, 147.

GRANICK, RUTH, and ZEMAN, F. D. (1960) The aged recluse—an exploratory study with special reference to community responsibility, *J. chron. Dis.*, **12**, 639.

GREWELL, F. (1953) Testing psychology of dementias, *Fol. psychiat. Neerl.*, **56**, 305.

GRUENTHAL, E. (1927) Klinisch-anatomisch vergleichende Untersuchungen ueber den Greisenbloedsinn, *Z. ges. Neurol. Psychiat.*, **111**, 763.

HAMILTON, L. D. and BENNETT, J. L. (1962) The use of trifluoperazine in geriatric patients with chronic brain syndrome, *J. Amer. Geriat. Soc.*, **10**, 140.

HILL, D. and DRIVER, M. V. (1962) in *Recent Advances in Neurology and Neuropsychiatry*, 7th Ed., Lord Brain, ed., J. & A. Churchill, London.

HIMWICH, A. WILHELMINA (1962) Neurochemistry of ageing, *Postgrad. Med.*, **31**, 195.

HIMWICH, WILHELMINA A. and HIMWICH, H. E. (1959) Neurochemistry of ageing, in Birren J. E. (ed.), *Handbook of Ageing and the Individual*, University of Chicago Press.

HIMWICH, H. E. (1962) Research in medical aspects of ageing, *Geriatrics*, **17**, 89.

HINTON, J. M. (1963) The physical and mental distress of the dying, *Quart. J. Med.*, **32**, 1.

HIRSCHMANN, J. (1962) Zur Kriminologie der Sexualdelikte des alternden Mannes, *Geront. Clin. Addiment*, 115.

HIRSCHMANN, J. and KLAGES, W. (1957) Konstitutionsspezifische Leitlinien bei den Psychosen des hoeheren Lebensalters, *Arch. f. Psychiat. & Zschr. f.d. ges. Neurol.*, **196**. 254

HOPKINS, BARBARA, and POST, F. (1955) The significance of abstract and concrete behaviour in elderly psychiatric patients and control subjects, *J. Ment. Sci.*, **101**, 841.

HOUSTON, F. and ROYSE, A. B. (1954) Relationship between deafness and psychotic illness, *J. Ment. Sci.*, **100**, 990.

INGLIS, J. (1957) An experiment of learning and "memory function" in elderly psychiatric patients, *J. Ment. Sci.*, **103**, 796.

INGLIS, J. (1958) Psychological investigations of cognitive deficit in elderly psychiatric patients, *Psychol. Bull.*, **55**, 197.

INGLIS, J., COLWELL, CATHERINE, and POST, F. (1960) An evaluation of the predictive power of a test known to differentiate between elderly "functional" and "organic" psychiatric patients, *J. Ment. Sci.*, **106**, 1486.

JANZARIK, W. (1957) Zur Problematik schizophrener Psychosen im höheren Lebensalter, *Nervenarzt*, **28**, 535.

JELGERSMA, H. C. (1958) Die fruehzeitige Dementia senilis bei Mongoloiden, *Fol. Psychiat. Neurol. Neerland.*, **61**, 367.

JONES, H. E. (1957) Age Changes in Mental Abilities in *Old Age in the Modern World*, Internat. Assoc. of Gerontology, London.

JONES, H. E. and KAPLAN, D. J. (1956) Psychological Aspects of Mental Disorders in Later Life in *Mental Disorders in Later Life*, Kaplan, D. J. (ed.), Stanford University Press.

KAHN, R. L., ZEMAN, F. D., and GOLDFARB, A. I. (1958) Attitudes towards illness in the aged, *Geriatrics*, **13**, 246.

KALLMANN, F. J. (1957) Twin Data on the Genetics of Ageing in *Ciba Foundation Colloquia on Ageing*, III, J. & A. Churchill, London.

KALLMANN, F. J. (1961) Genetic Factors in Ageing: Comparative and longitudinal Observations on a senescent Twin Population, in *Psychopathology of Ageing*, Hoch, P. H. and Zubin, J. (eds.), Grune & Stratton, New York.

KATZ, L., NEAL, M. W., and SIMON, A. (1961) Observations on psychic mechanisms in organic psychoses of the aged in *Psychopathology of Ageing*, Hoch, P. H. and Zubin, J. (eds.), Grune & Stratton, New York.

KAY, D. W. K. (1959) Observations on the natural history and genetics of old age psychoses: A Stockholm material, 1931–1937, *Proc. Roy. Soc. Med.*, **52**, 791.

KAY, D. W. K., ROTH, M., HOPKINS, BARBARA (1955) Affective Disorders in the Senium: (1) Their association with organic cerebral degeneration, *J. Ment. Sci.*, **101**, 302.

KAY, D. W. K., and ROTH, M. (1961) Environmental and hereditary factors in the schizophrenias of old age ("Late Paraphrenia") and their bearing on the general problem of causation in schizophrenia, *J. Ment. Sci.*, **107**, 649.

KENDALL, BARBARA S. (1962) Memory-for-designs performance in the seventh and eighth decades of life, *Percept. Mot. Skills*, **14**, 399.

KENDRICK, D. C., PARBOOSINGH, R. CECILE, and POST, F. (1963) In preparation.

KENNEDY, A. (1959) Psychological factors in confusional states in the elderly, *Geront. Clin.*, **1**, 71.

KESSEL, N. and SHEPHERD, M. (1962) Neurosis in hospital and general practice, *J. Ment. Sci.*, **108**, 159.

KINSEY, A. C., POMEROY, W. B., and MARTIN, C. E. (1948) *Sexual Behaviour in the Human Male*, W. B. Saunders & Co., Philadelphia.

KINSEY, A. C., POMEROY, W. B., MARTIN, C. E., and GEBHARD, P. M. (1953) *Sexual Behaviour in the Human Female*, W. B. Saunders & Co., Philadelphia.

KOLLE, K. (1931) *Die primaere Verruecktheit*, Georg Thieme, Leipzig.

KRAL, V. A. (1962) Senescent forgetfulness: Benign and malignant, *Canad. Med. Ass. J.*, **86**, 257.

LANGFELDT, G. (1960) Diagnosis and prognosis of schizophrenia, *Proc. Roy. Soc. Med.*, **53**, 1047.

LARSSON, T., SJOEGREN, T., and JACOBSON, G. (1963) Senile Dementia, *Act. Psychiat. Scand.*, **39**, Supp. 167.

LASSEN, N. H., FEINBERG, I., and LANE, M. H. (1960) Bilateral studies of cerebral oxygen uptake in young and aged normal subjects and in patients with organic dementia, *J. Clin. Invest.*, **39**, 491.

LECHLER, H. (1950) Die Psychosen der Alten, *Arch. Psychiat. Nervenkr.*, **185**, 465.

LEWIS, A. (1955) Mental Aspects of Ageing, *Ciba Foundation Coll. Ageing*, **1**, 32, Churchill, London.

LINDEN, M. E. (1953) Group psychotherapy with institutionalised senile women, *Internat. J. Group Psychotherapy*, **3**, 150.

LLEWELLYN, A. (1961) Management of confusion and restlessness in the aged, *Brit. J. Clin. Pract.*, **15**, 839.

LORGE, S. and TUCKMAN, J. (1953) *Retirement and the Industrial Worker*, Columbia University Press, New York.

McCORMICK, W. O. (1962) *A Study of the Relationship between Dementia and radiologically diagnosed Cerebral Atrophy in elderly Patients*, Diss. for the Academ. Postgrad. Diploma in Psychological Medicine, Institute of Psychiatry, London.

McMENEMY, W. N., GREENFIELD, J. G., BLACKWOOD, W., MEYER, A. and NORMAN, R. M. (1958) *Neuropathology*, Edward Arnold, London.

MACMILLAN, D. (1960) Preventive geriatrics, *Lancet*, II, 1439.

MAYER-GROSS, W. (1932) Schizophrenie, Bumke's Handbuch der Geisteskrankheiten, Spec. Pt. 5, Chapts. IV and V., Springer, Berlin.

MEAD, B. T. (1962) Emotional struggles in adjusting to old age, *Postgrad. Med.*, **31**, 156.

MEDAWAR, P. B. (1957) *The Uniqueness of the Individual*, Methuen, London.

MEERLOO, J. A. M. (1955) Transference and resistance in geriatric psychotherapy, *Psychoanalyt. Rev.*, **42**.

Mental Health Research Unit, New York, State Department of Mental Hygiene, (1960/61) *A Mental Health Survey of Older People*, State Hospitals Press, Utica, N.Y.

MILLER, H. C. (1963) *The Ageing Countryman*, National Corporation for the Care of Old People, London.

MITCHELL, JOYCE (1958) Speech and language impairment in the older patient. Some problems in management, *Geriatrics*, **13**, 467.

MITCHELL, J. M. (1957) An hypothesis of psychological ageing, *Amer. J. Psychol.*, **70**, 459.

MUELLER, C. (1953) Vorlaeufige Mitteilung zur langen Katamnese der Zwangskranken, *Nervenarzt.*, **24**, 112.

MUELLER, C. (1959) *Ueber das Senium der Schizophrenen*, S. Karger, Basel.

MUNNICHS, J. M. A. (1961) Comments at the symposium on attitudes towards death in older persons, *J. Gerontol.*, **16**, 60.

NEWMAN, G. and NICHOLLS, C. R. (1960) Sexual activities and attitudes in older persons, *J.A.M.A.*, **173**, 33.

NORRIS, VERA (1959) *Mental Illness in London*, Maudsley Monograph No. 6, Institute of Psychiatry, London.

OAKLEY, D. P. (1962) *The Aetiology of Senile Dementia*, Unpublished M.D. Thesis, University of Manchester.

PAMPIGLIONE, G. and POST, F. (1958) The value of electroencephalographic examination in psychiatric disorders of old age, *Geriatrics*, **13**, 725.

PARSONS, P. N. (1962) *The Health of Swansea's Old Folk: A Survey of a Random Sample of the Elderly living in their own Homes*, Unpublished M.D. Thesis, University of Wales.

POST, F. (1944) Some problems arising from a study of mental patients over the age of sixty years, *J. Ment. Sci.*, **90**, 554.

POST, F. (1959) Early treatment of persistent senile confusion, *Geront. Clin.*, **1**, 114.

POST, F. (1962) *The Significance of Affective Symptoms in Old Age*, Maudsley Monograph, **10**, Oxford University Press.

POST, F. (1962) The Impact of modern drug treatment on Old Age Schizophrenia, *Geront. Clin.*, **4**, 137.

POST, F. (1962) The social orbit of psychiatric patients, *J. Ment. Sci.*, **108**, 759.

RAVEN, J. C. (1958a) *Guide to using The Mill Hill Vocabulary Scale with the Progressive Matrices*, H. K. Lewis, London.

RAVEN, J. C. (1958b) *Guide to using the Coloured Progressive Matrices*, H. K. Lewis, London.

RECHTSCHAFFEN, A. (1959) Psychotherapy with geriatric patients: A review of the literature, *J. Gerontol.*, **14**, 73.

RECHTSCHAFFEN, A., ATKINSON, S., and FREEMAN, J. G. (1953) An intensive treatment program for state hospital geriatric patients, *Geriatrics*, **9**, 28.

REICHARD, SUZANNE, LIVSON, FLORINE, and PETERSON, P. G. (1962) *Ageing and Personality*, John Wiley & Sons, New York.

REMY, M. (1962) Emploi prolongé des neuroleptiques en psychiatrie, *Praxis (Rev. Suisse Med.)*, **11**, 288.

RICHARDSON, I. M. (1956) Retirement, A socio-medical study of 244 men, *Scot. M.J.*, **1**, 381.

ROSEN, G. (1961) Cross-cultural and historical Approaches in *Psychopathology of Ageing*, Hoch, P. H. and Zubin, J. (eds.), Grune & Stratton, New York.

ROTH, M. (1955) The natural history of mental disorder in old age, *J. Ment. Sci.*, **101**, 281.

ROTHSCHILD, D. (1937) Pathologic changes in senile psychoses and their psychobiologic significance, *Amer. J. Psychiat.*, **93**, 757.

ROTHSCHILD, D. (1942) Neuropathological changes in arteriosclerotic psychosis and their psychiatric significance, *Arch. Neurol. Psychiat. (Chicago)*, **48**, 417.

ROTHSCHILD, D. (1956) Senile Psychoses and Psychoses with Cerebral Arteriosclerosis in *Mental Disorders in Later Life*, Kaplan, O. J. (ed.), Stanford University Press, Stanford.

SAINSBURY, P. (1962) Suicide in later life, *Geront. Clin.*, **4**, 161.

SANDERSON, R. E. and INGLIS, J. (1961) Learning and mortality in elderly psychiatric patients, *J. Gerontol.*, **16**, 375.

SAVITSKY, E. (1953) Psychological factors in nutrition of the aged, *Social Case Work*, Dec.

SCHNEIDER, K. (1955) *Klinische Psychopathologie*, Georg Thieme, Stuttgart.

SHAPIRO, M. B., FIELD, J., and POST, F. (1957) An enquiry into the determinants of a differentiation between elderly "organic" and "non-organic" psychiatric patients on the Bender Gestalt Test, *J. Ment. Sci.*, **103**, 364.

SHAPIRO, M. B. and NELSON, E. H. (1955) An Investigation of the nature of cognitive impairment in co-operative psychiatric patients, *Brit. J. Med. Psychol.*, **28**, 239.

SHAPIRO, M. B., POST, F., LOEFVING, BARBRO, and INGLIS, J. (1956) "Memory function" in psychiatric patients over 60; some methodological and diagnostic implications, *J. Ment. Sci.*, **106**, 223.

SHELDON, J. H. (1948) *The Social Medicine of Old Age*. Oxford University Press. London.

SHOCK, N. W. (1961) Current concepts of the ageing process, *J.A.M.A.*, **175**, 654.

SHOCK, N. W. (1963) *A Classified Bibliography of Gerontology and Geriatrics*, Stanford University Press, Stanford.

SILVER, A. (1950) Group psychotherapy with senile psychotic women, *Geriatrics*, **5**, 147.

SILVERMAN, A. J., BUSSE, E. W., and BARNES, R. (1955) Studies in the processes of ageing: Electroencephalographic findings in 400 elderly subjects, *EEG. Clin. Neurophysiol.*, **7**, 67.

SJOEGREN, T., SJOEGREN, H., and LINDGREN, A. G. H. (1952) *Morbus Alzheimer and Morbus Pick*, *Act. Psychiat. Neurol. Scand.*, Supp. 82.

SLATER, E., BEARD, A. W., and CLITHERO, E. (1963) The schizophrenic-like psychoses of epilepsy, *Brit. J. Psychiat.*, **109**, 95.

SOURS, J. A. (1960) Some neurologic and psychiatric aspects of bilateral internal carotid occlusion: A case report, *J. Ment. Sci.*, **106**, 1063.

STENSTEDT, A. (1959) *Involutional Melancholia*, *Act. Psychiat. Neurol. Scand.* Supp. 127.

STERN, K. (1957) Reactive Depressions in Late Life in *Depression*, Hoch, P. H. and Zubin, J. (eds.), Grune & Stratton, New York.

SZILLARD, L. (1959) A theory of ageing, *Nature*, **184**, 956.

TALLAND, G. A. and CLARK, D. H. (1954) Evaluation of topics in therapy and group discussion, *J. Clin. Psychol.*, **10**, 131.

THOMPSON, W. E. and SUCHMAN, E. A. (1958) The Cornell Study of occupational retirement, *J. of Social Issues*, **14**, 3.

THORPE, F. T. (1958) An evaluation of prefrontal leucotomy in the affective disorders of old age: A follow-up study, *J. Ment. Sci.*, **104**, 403.

THORPE, F. T. (1960) Electrocoagulation of the cerebral orbital projection in the persistent depressive psychoses of the elderly, *J. Ment. Sci.*, **106**, 771.

TOWNSEND, P. (1957) *The Family Life of Old People*, Routledge & Kegan Paul, London.

TOWNSEND, P. (1962) *The Last Refuge. A Survey of Residential Institutions and Homes for the Aged in England and Wales*, Routledge & Kegan Paul, London.

TURTON, E. C. (1958) The EEG as a diagnostic and prognostic aid in the differentiation of organic disorders in patients over 60, *J. Ment. Sci.*, **104**, 461.

VERZÁR, F. (1957) Studies in adaptation as a method of gerontological research, *Ciba Found. Coll. Ageing*, *III*, 159, Churchill, London.

VERZÁR-MCDOUGALL, E. J. (1957) Studies in learning and memory in ageing rats, *Gerontologia*, **1**, 67.

WAHAL, K. M. and RIGGS, HELENA E. (1960) Changes in the brain associated with Senility, *A.M.A. Arch. Neurol.*, **2**, 151.

WALTON, D. (1958) The diagnostic and predictive accuracy of the modified word learning test in psychiatric patients over 65, *J. Ment. Sci.*, **104**, 1119.

WALTON, D. and BLACK, D. A. (1957) The validity of a psychological test of brain damage, *Brit. J. Med. Psychol.*, **30**, 270.

WAYNE, G. J. (1952) Psychotherapy in Senescence, *Amer. West. Med. & Surg.*, **6**, 88.

WEATHERALL, M. (1962) Tranquillisers, *Brit. Med. J.*, **1**, 1219.

WECHSLER, D. (1961) Intelligence, Memory and the Ageing Process in *Psychopathology of Ageing*, Hoch, P. H. and Zubin, J. (eds.), Grune & Stratton, New York.

WELFORD, A. T. (1958) Psychological and social gerontology in Europe, *J. Gerontol.*, **13**, 51.

WELFORD, A. T. (1962) On changes of performance with age, *The Lancet*, **1**, 335.

WILLIAMS, H. W., QUESNEL, E., FISH, V. W., and GOODMAN, L. (1942) Studies in senile and arteriosclerotic psychoses, *Amer. J. Psychiat.*, **98**, 712.

WILLIAMS, MOYRA (1956) Studies of perception in senile dementia: Cue-selection as a function of intelligence, *Brit. J. Med. Psychol.*, **29**, 270.

WILLMOTT, P. and YOUNG, M. (1960) *Family and Class in a London Suburb*, Routledge & Kegan Paul, London.

WILSON, L. A. and LAWSON, I. R. (1962) Situational depression in the elderly: A study of 23 cases, *Geront. Clin.*, *Addit. ad Vol. 4*, 59.

WOLFF, K. (1963) *Geriatric Psychiatry*, Thomas, Springfield.

YATES, A. J. (1954) The validity of some psychological tests of brain damage, *Psychol. Bull.*, **51**, 359.

ZEMAN, F. D. (1962) Pathologic anatomy of old age, *A.M.A. Arch. Path.*, **73**, 126.

INDEX

171

POST: Clinical psychiatry of late life